After studying biological medicine at the Heilpraktikerssc ule in Solingen in Germany (1977), **Jan Dries** speciali: d in nutritional therapy in association with the Avicenna Health Centre in Genk. Since then he has met and worked with thousands of people in search of a better diet.

A lecturer at the Academy of Natural Medicine in Bloemendaal and Amsterdam, Holland for eight years, Jan Dries has since 1988 been the chairman of the Executive Board of the European Academy of Complementary Medicine in Antwerp and Ghent (Belgium) and Utrecht and Maastricht (Holland). He is also chairman of the Vegetarian Society and the New Life Society, and founder of the Association of Naturopaths; and he holds distinguished offices in a number of other associations.

Previously published works include 35 books and more than a hundred pamphlets on the subject of health, all of which have achieved some repute. In addition to his painstaking research in the field of nutrition, he has also made important contributions to such disciplines as bio-energy, herbal and natural medicine, relaxation therapy and reflexology.

Over the past five years he has treated more than 600 cancer patients with his 'Dries cancer diet', a method that has gained him international renown. As an experienced nutritionist who has guided cancer patients on their way to a healthy diet, Jan Dries has written his book drawing upon his ample experience. He not only elaborates upon the practical application of the diet named after him, but also stresses the benefit of a number of other complementary therapies.

Dr Sandra Goodman, a molecular biology scientist, has written four books on nutritional subjects, including two about nutrition and cancer. She set up the Nutrition and Cancer Database, containing over 3,000 records, for the Bristol Cancer Help Centre. She is the publisher of *Positive Health* magazine, a serious publication about the entire spectrum of complementary therapies, and can be contacted at the address given at the back of this book.

by the same author

The New Book of Food Combining

also available

200 New Food Combining Recipes: Tasty Dishes from Around the World by Inge Dries

---

Important Information

- The Dries cancer diet is meant to complement and to support regular treatment.

- The diet is not suitable for diabetics or for patients who are not allowed to use sugar or who are only allowed to use a limited amount of sugar.

- The diet is not suitable for people who suffer from anorexia or malnourishment.

- When in doubt or in case of problems, contact your doctor immediately.

- Professional advice and counselling are recommended.

- The Author and the Publisher are not responsible for the possible results of incorrect application of the diet or for failure to obtain results by means of the diet.

The Dries Cancer Diet

A PRACTICAL GUIDE TO
THE USE OF FRESH FRUIT
AND RAW VEGETABLES IN THE
TREATMENT OF CANCER

JAN DRIES

ELEMENT

Shaftesbury, Dorset • Rockport, Massachusetts • Melbourne, Victoria

© Element Books Limited 1997
Text © Jan Dries 1997

First published in Dutch under the title *Er is Nog Hoop, als Kanker Toeslaat*
Uitgeverij Arinus Belgium

First published in Great Britain in 1997 by
Element Books Limited
Shaftesbury, Dorset SP7 8BP

Published in the USA in 1997 by
Element Books, Inc.
PO Box 830, Rockport, MA 01966

Published in Australia in 1997 by 2/98
Element Books
and distributed by Penguin Australia Ltd
487 Maroondah Highway, Ringwood, Victoria 3134

Design by Roger Lightfoot
Typeset by Footnote Graphics
Printed and bound in Great Britain by
J. W. Arrowsmith, Bristol

British Library Cataloguing in Publication data available

Library of Congress Cataloging in Publication data available

ISBN 1–85204–092–3

Contents

List of Figures

Foreword

That diet plays an important role in preventing many types of cancer is documented repeatedly in an ever-burgeoning body of international scientific research, published throughout the past several decades. As a scientist who has waded through thousands of such research studies in order to compile a research database about Nutrition and Cancer, I have often been amazed at the general lack of awareness and acknowledgement, from maintstream medical practitioners and oncologists, of this research performed by the world's leading epidemiologists, clinicians and oncologists and published in the most prestigious peer-reviewed learned journals.

Study after study affirms that people who eat more fruits and vegetables, less fat and more fibre, and who have higher blood plasma levels of antioxidant nutrients including beta carotene, vitamins A, C, E and selenium are at significantly reduced risks of having many kinds of cancer, as well as other major conditions such as heart disease. Recent examples include a study from New York State (*J Nat Cancer Inst* 88(6): 340–8, 20 March 1996) which found that the risk of breast cancer in premenopausal women was significantly reduced – 0.46–0.67 – in those women with the highest intake of vitamins C, E, alpha- and beta-carotene and dietary fibre from vegetable and fruits. There was a strong inverse association found between risk and total vegetable intake, although no association between risk and intake of these vitamins taken as supplements. This kind of research results, which have been replicated in many large-scale studies in many parts of the world, have led international government bodies to advise their populations to consume at least five servings of fruits and vegetables per day.

However, although certain nutrients appear to offer significant protection against cancer, this does not prove that people get cancer because they have or have not eaten these foods. Epidemiology is a science which provides statistical odds ratios, not direct causal links. This is where clinical scientists have stepped in, working with nutrients to treat cancer, in studies with cells, animals and human subjects. There have been many published studies with a variety of nutrients – Vitamins A, C, E, selenium, beta-carotene and essential fatty acids – and their effects in treating a variety of cancers.

Researchers investigating the mode of action of certain nutrients toward cancer cells, including antioxidants and essential fatty acids, have found that these nutrients are cytotoxic – that is, can kill or disrupt the activity of cancerous cells. Research at the molecular and biochemical levels is focused at discovering how certain nutrients act at the molecular level to modulate the activity of certain cancer genes. Nutrients such as beta-carotene, lycopene, omega-3 fatty acids and polyphenols in wine are the subject of intense research interest. One study from Israel (*Nutr Cancer* 24(3): 257–66, 1995) showed that lycopene, the major carotenoid from tomato, strongly inhibited the proliferation of endometrial, mammary and lung human cancer cells and was a more effective inhibitor of human cancer cell growth than alpha- and beta-carotene. The research continues.

Almost everyone, including Jan Dries, agrees that cancer is an extremely unpredictable disease and that its behaviour, unfortunately, is unique for each individual. There are no firm certainties, regardless of the course of treatment followed, of who will survive and who will not. This applies to people whose cancer is treated with surgery, chemotherapy and radiotherapy, as well as those incorporating alternative treatments with diet, visualization and other 'lifestyle change' approaches.

The Dries diet is based largely upon the consumption of raw

fruits, most prominently of tropical fruit such as pineapple and mango, as well as certain raw vegetables, seeds, and condiments such as yoghurt, buttermilk and some oils. The basis of the selection of these foods is their bio-energetic value measured in biophotons which apparently has an effect upon resistance to cancer. This kind of research is quite novel, so that it is difficult for me to judge its validity. Nevertheless, I am genuinely interested in the results which Jan Dries is obtaining with his patients, who are also receiving mainstream medical treatment.

Unlike many other proponents of special cancer diets, Jan Dries is refreshingly humble and acknowledges the impossibility of predicting the outcome of cancer and encourages his patients to follow treatment advised by their doctors. His discussion of resultant amelioration of side-effects achieved by this diet, and sometimes of complete recovery, merit the attention and respect of cancer specialists, even if they can't accept or understand why the diet appears to work. Jan Dries describes some of the pitfalls and side-effects encountered by patients who launch into the diet 'cold turkey', provides practical tips about how to implement the diet, including shopping lists and menus, and includes an array of personal case histories, incorporating some of his own observations about why there has been such an increase in the incidence of cancer.

There are many special diets for cancer, including raw foods, cooked foods and mixtures thereof; each of these regimes claims successes in some instances. Nobody to my knowledge has yet discovered a universal cure for cancer and, until they do, it is the responsibility of every physician and researcher to investigate and reserve judgement upon regimes until their worth is either proven or disproven.

Thus a book such as this one by Jan Dries, who has been working successfully with cancer patients for many years, needs to be read not only by cancer patients but by the wider medical community at large, despite the scepticism they may have about the particulars of this diet. Could it be that these particular fruits have some cytotoxic effect upon cancer cells, or that consuming a diet of mainly raw fruit allows the body to detoxify, and enables the immune system to fight the cancer? Or both? It is my fervent hope that research in the very near future can tackle this kind of nutritional question relating to cancer. In the meantime, I also hope that Jan Dries's diet will be the subject of intense scrutiny, debate and interest among the medical community and among cancer sufferers.

Sandra Goodman, PhD.

Preface

It is remarkable that no new cancer diets have been developed since the 1950s. Regular cancer *treatment* has been given prominence for many years: new research techniques, accurate surgery, improved chemotherapy and more precisely dosed amounts of radiation have given new hope. Because of all that, the *biological fight against* cancer has been completely forgotten. But in spite of those positive developments the cancer problem is still growing. The number of adults and children suffering from cancer is still increasing. Brain tumours occur more frequently than before. Cancer seems to spread more rapidly these days and relapse is not at all out of the ordinary. We have lost control over the cancer problem and most people fear the situation will only become worse.

The cancer problem has been lifted out of its narrow medical context. After all, it is a very complicated disease. Cancer is a social problem that is closely related to a materialistic way of life, environmental pollution, stress, emotional disorders and especially food. It is the job of the doctors to apply medical treatments and to guide cancer patients medically, but correctly. It contains examples of recovery cases and practical tips. Many aspects of cancer will be discussed, although the keynote throughout this book will be food. This book results from my ample experience with food therapy and my daily contact with cancer patients, with whose painful and persistent agony I am very familiar. The promise of this book lies in the fact that it offers something very ordinary, something that is part of daily life: food. Everyone can apply this diet as a supplement to his or her regular treatment. The diet holds no dangers and there are absolutely no side-effects. It does on the other hand increase chances of recovery and strongly reduce the side-effects of regular treatments. Those who read this book should be convinced of the fact that food and lifestyle are very important, both for the prevention of cancer and for supporting the recovery from cancer. Many forms of support are needed, especially those afforded by complementary treatments.

I was one of the first people to start researching into complementary cancer treatment. Unlike many pioneers of the biological fight against cancer who completely rejected regular treatment, my work was designed to complement it. After years of intensive experimentation, I have systematically composed the diet that bears my name. Now that I believe the success of the Dries diet can no longer be doubted, I wish to introduce my diet to a wider audience through this book.

This book describes the relationship of food and cancer, examines the bio-energetic aspect of this relationship, explains the composition of the diet and teaches everyone how to apply the diet supporting the recovery from cancer. I also give much attention to the importance of relaxation therapy. Good relaxation influences not only the effects of the diet but also the overall condition of the patient.

This book should convince everyone who reads it, because it gives acceptable answers to many questions that are asked regarding the subjects of food and cancer. It had a scientific basis, although in it I have deliberately chosen not to pursue scientific discussions. I have tried to write an accessible and useful book, a book whose message is heartfelt, and I hope that that in itself will mean something to most people.

Introduction

The introduction of an article or a book about cancer nearly always confronts us with a spectre of the disease. It usually evokes images of the approaching end. All we an read about is 'the merciless usurper', 'the horrible disease' and the risk of dying. I would like to introduce this book in a completely different way, because there is still hope in spite of everything. We have to learn how to see cancer differently. We have to deal with cancer in a different way and find the courage to turn to alternative therapeutic possibilities.

In this book, my principal theme will be the favourable influence of certain kinds of food. Which foodstuffs I am talking about and how to use them will be explained by means of a diet that bears my name: the Dries diet. For many years, this diet has been successfully applied by hundreds of cancer patients, whether or not under my supervision. Many patients, their relatives and their attending physicians acknowledge the influence of my cancer diet.

Numerous scientific studies have provided us with irrefutable evidence showing that an industrialized feeding pattern has a lot of influence on the development of cancer. Luckily, more and more people are starting to think in a positive way. They realize that vegetarian food can slow cancer down. The most important thing in the fight against cancer is the way in which we think about cancer. As long as we do not work on changing that aspect, the reign of terror will not diminish . . . on the contrary: consider the following example.

One day a man was told he had cancer. The little hope he had managed to hang on to in spite of presentiments was immediately crushed. To get rid of his restlessness he went for a walk in his neighbourhood. Simply because he was bored or angry, he picked a flower that was growing by the roadside. Despairing and speechless, he looked at the flower between his trembling fingers. For the first time in his life, he was really looking at a flower and it suddenly started to fascinate him. At that ultimate moment he discovered the coherence in life. He found the way to nature, our origin. The incident changed his life completely. He started to think differently about life and about the illness he was suffering from. What is cancer? How does it start? Why do people get cancer? These are all questions nobody – not even an oncologist – can answer. What we do know – and this is very important – is that cancer is a disease of civilization. The more man becomes separated from nature, the more likely he is to get cancer. That man's flower and its indescribable beauty gave him the go-ahead for gaining new insight into this terrible disease. The greatest wisdom and the ultimate healing power are to be found in nature. Hippocrates already said it 2,500 years ago: 'Not the doctor, but nature heals.'

I have guided hundreds of cancer patients on their way to a healthy diet. Many of them had been told by their physicians that they had no chance of recovery, but they recovered anyway, against all odds. People with metastasis in lungs, liver and bones recovered quite quickly. Unfortunately I was not able to help everyone. In some patients the illness was already so far advanced that there was no way back. But even those patients were able to lengthen their lives and especially improve the quality of their lives, even in such a way that medical care could be reduced to a minimum. All these results were diagnosed by physicians and by the patients themselves. Most physicians were baffled by the remarkable results. They could not believe their own eyes when they saw the results and yet in most cases they had to admit that the Dries diet was the decisive factor. Food therapy is completely unknown in regular medicine, which is exactly the reason why some people do not know what to do with it.

In this book, I do not wish to provoke bombastic discussions or theories. I only want to point out that – apart from necessary surgery, chemotherapy or radiation treatment – the Dries diet can be an important complementary therapy. The Dries diet increases the chance of recovery and reduces the side-effects of the therapies mentioned earlier. Based on my experience, I cannot stress strongly enough the necessity of the diet. On the other hand I understand that it is not always easy to move on to a diet that thoroughly differs from traditional eating habits. And I have not yet mentioned the vital support of the relatives or the physician.

This book is the product of years of experience. I know the difficulties cancer patients have to deal with. That is exactly why I want to stress the practical application of my diet. Furthermore, I wish to urge readers to use my diet, which they will only do if I can prove the value of the diet and eliminate doubts. My aim is to do that by means of scientific data and reflection based on very recent literature. Never forget that we will not gain any insight unless we let ourselves be stimulated by the wisdom of mother nature. Both cancer research and cancer treatment are dominated by the medical–technical aspect, which is understandable if you know that time plays a very important part in cases of cancer. If you want to save a human life, you have to intervene rapidly and use radical means to do so. But there is more to cancer than just the medical–technical aspect. Cancer is enclosed by humanity and the more unnatural a society's lifestyle, the more likely it is to occur. That is the principle I would like to start from in this book and that is the way in which I would like my diet to be considered. Nevertheless, it is extremely important not to lose sight of the powerful effects or the many favourable results of the diet.

I believe in miracles because I have seen so many of them happen. That is why I can say with conviction: there is still hope.

Chapter 1

Cancer: a Brief Description

The famous German pathologist Prof. Dr Bier (1861–1949) once said: 'You can easily fill a whole library with articles on the subject cancer, but everything we actually know about cancer would barely fill a business card.' Ever since this famous statement was made, many articles about cancer have been published. There is no doubt that we have been able to gain much knowledge over the years. Every year, vast amounts of money are spent on cancer research. Unfortunately cancer research has not been able to make any concrete progress yet. Of course it is more or less generally known how cancer develops – that a tumour grows, that cell division (fission) takes place and that the tumour spreads (metastasis); a cell becomes a cancer cell when wrong information is passed. We have discovered onco-genes and proto-oncogenes as well as oncoplacentary proteins, cancer antigens, etc. We also know a great deal about mutation. There has been remarkable progress in genetics over the past few years, and there is obviously no lack of scientific data; nobody questions the benefit of the knowledge we have. But all research thus far has been relatively unsuccessful because the number of cancer cases is still increasing at an alarming rate. The risk of getting cancer and dying of it increases every day. Statistics indicate that – within the European Union – 2,500 people are diagnosed with cancer every day. In spite of apparent success with some forms of treatment, cancer still remains a serious problem. The statistics seem to show that the increase in cancer cases runs parallel to the ageing of the population. And indeed it is true that cancer occurs more frequently in older people than it does in younger people. As the number of elderly increases, the number of cancer patients belonging to that group also increases; but that should not be the decisive factor when we study the general increase in numbers of cancer cases. In spite of scientific research, massive education, large-scale national research, improved methods of diagnosis, adapted treatments and especially the major involvement of every individual involved in the campaign against cancer, we still find the number of people suffering from cancer increases by 2–3 per cent every year.

Cancer is and remains a little understood disease, which is especially due to the fact that cancer originates at cellular level. Cancer is invisible. It strikes without warning. It does not possess any early tell-tale characteristics and it only reveals itself in the critical phase. It is often rightly said that cancer is not really a disease in a conventional sense, because it is unlike any other disease. Even the development of the tumour goes by unnoticed, painless and without influencing the general health of the victim. Many cancer patients have told me: 'I feel excellent and I can handle all kinds of work. I don't believe I have cancer.' It seems as if cancer exists independent of the human, but once the disease is present, it takes over the whole body by means of festering growth. If cancer is not treated in time, the effects within a few years are devastating. Almost all organs become affected and bones become brittle. Finally, the human body turns into a culture medium for the tumour or tumours. The body's resources are completely used up, until the vital organs are affected and death occurs. Expressions like 'the merciless usurper' or 'the sly murderer' are definitely appropriate here.

Cancer in itself is a painless disease, but that is exactly what makes it so insidious. That cancer is painless is understandable, for a tumour is in fact nothing but tissue consisting of cells. The only difference between a healthy cell and a cancer cell is in their behaviour. Pain is a warning sign, an unpleasant sensation that forces us to react; but because a tumour does not hurt, we cannot react to it. And even if a tumour presses against an organ, a nerve, a muscle or certain tissue, the body will react to that pressure only, not to the tumour itself. Most of the time, secondary pain signals are of such nature that we immediately pay a visit to our GP. Once the tumour starts its destructive work, the body reacts to that. But unfortunately that means the disease has already reached an advanced stage. Only tumours that are located on the surface of the body can be detected by chance or by means of precautionary examination. Deep (well-hidden) tumours – such as tumours in the brain, stomach, intestines, kidneys or lungs – are virtually never discovered early. Once the disease cancer is inside the body, it causes the cells to mutate and create a tumour. The disease is already present prior to the tumour's development.

Because cancer is an invisible disease, all cancer research is still an uphill battle. We can only take action when the tumour has already revealed itself. Research can only examine tumours, and tumours are just symptoms of the disease. A tumour barely leaves traces in the blood and in other bodily fluids. Tumour markers are not cell-specific products. They are substances that are also secreted by benign or normal cells. That is why they do not have a decisive meaning for the diagnosis and certainly not for precautionary examination. Tumour markers do say something about the seriousness of the matter though, and they can be used to follow the evolution of the tumour. The disease itself cannot be examined and therefore remains the great unknown.

We tend to talk about cancer only when there is a tumour. If that is not the case, but there are signs that a tumour may develop, we talk about a precancerous stage. When someone is still in a precancerous stage, for example, we can discover tissue changes that may degenerate, or atypical cell multiplications that have a certain tendency to exceed the physiological boundaries of a tissue. Such cells are called 'agitated/restless' cells. The disease has not manifested itself yet and for the time being there

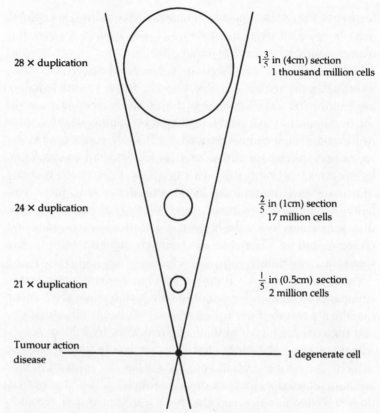

28 × duplication

$1\frac{3}{5}$ in (4cm) section
1 thousand million cells

24 × duplication

$\frac{2}{5}$ in (1cm) section
17 million cells

21 × duplication

$\frac{1}{5}$ in (0.5cm) section
2 million cells

Tumour action
disease

1 degenerate cell

Figure 1 *Diagram of incipient cancer and the development of a tumour*

is no immediate danger. A precancerous stage can be treated quite easily. The question is whether or not the patient already has cancer at this stage. The answer is ambiguous. If we consider the risk and the prospects for treatment we can safely say that someone in a precancerous stage does not have cancer yet. But from the aetiological point of view this is not the case. A tumour cannot develop if there is no cancer. Cancer is a pathological condition that may involve the development of tumours. Regular research and treatment both concentrate on the tumour. Surgically removing the tumour does not guarantee recovery from the cancer. Unfortunately, every day there are people who experience regression/relapse. There have been attempts to make cancer research concentrate more on incipient cancer, but current methods make that rather difficult.

Bio-energetic research on the other hand offers new possibilities. (In my book *Bio-energy, Our Life Force*, I give a complete description of what bio-energy is and how our daily lives can depend upon it. I will not be explaining it elaborately here, but I will be discussing its relevance to the Dries Cancer Diet.) When we start approaching illness and health from an bio-energetic perspective, we are dealing with invisible quantities and that is the most important factor. After all, cancer is caused by an energetic malfunction and manifests itself on that level. To stress the importance of bio-energetics, I will briefly explain the development of a cancer cell. Just like vegetable and animal organisms, the human organism is based on a genetic code that is located in the DNA of the cells. That genetic code can be compared to an extremely sophisticated computer system that is provided not only with all features but also with all signals that are necessary to make physiological and biochemical processes possible. When a cell divides itself, for example, it is decided which part of the code is needed, taking the other cells into account; this happens at the speed of light. A cell always has a very specific function in the organism. Malignant cells are produced in exactly the same way. The only difference is that we do not understand why they are produced. Some say it is because there is a defect; others claim it happens when the organism finds itself in a state of emergency and tries to find a way out by means of producing malignant cells. In the first case the question is why there is a defect. When the cancer is caused by an exogenous factor, it is obvious how it originates. Being exposed to a high dose of radioactivity or a high concentration of carcinogenic chemicals can cause our cells to mutate, in the same way that viruses do. But this question still remains unanswered: 'Why does this lead to cancer in one case and not in the other?' Every individual possesses a 'cancer resistance', a security system that is similar to the immune system.

The second argument – that is, that cancer is a way out, an attempt to prevent worse from happening – is similar to the theory of incapacity. It seems as if cancer patients are not capable of really becoming ill. It is remarkable that most cancer patients have never been ill before and have always been very healthy, even when the tumour was already present. Humoral pathology, based on the principles of Hippocrates, Galenus and Avincenna, claims that illness is caused by pollution of the bodily fluids. That is why some people believe that tumours develop in order to clear up toxic substances. Their theory is that cancer develops when the boundary of auto-intoxication is exceeded. Even though this theory seems very logical, it does raise some doubts, especially because it takes quite a long time for a tumour to reach its full growth. Moreover, the theory is not very clear regarding the destructive action of a tumour. It seems to claim that cancer is a disease that is inside our body like a kind of predestination.

Certain circumstances – both emotional and physiological – cause cancer to reveal itself. Extensive research shows that cancer often develops after a traumatic confrontation: the death of a loved one, a divorce, a severe disappointment, a prolonged stress situation, etc. Physiological circumstances such as, for example, a serious disease seldom lead to the development of cancer. Cancer more often develops in a healthy than in an unhealthy organ, although there are exceptions. Intestinal cancer, for example, may develop after a long history of intestinal disease, whereas stomach cancer may also develop in a stomach that has always been healthy. It is erroneous to claim that cancer always develops in a weak organ. In any case, cancer already develops long before the tumour becomes visible, and all this happens in the most mysterious circumstances: the development of cancer in the human body always goes by unnoticed. The origin of cancer still remains a mystery.

It is exactly because of its insidious nature that cancer is such an emotional disease. Talking about cancer is still considered a taboo by a lot of people. The cruel unpredictability of the disease, the aggressive treatments with uncertain results, the deterioration process and the suffering that nearly all cancer patients undergo make cancer so dreaded.

In order to start treatment, there has to be a tumour first. Medical science, including the field of oncology, is very advanced these days. But even the most sophisticated surgery is not good enough, because it is in fact nearly always performed too late. When a tumour is discovered, even in the early stages, the disease is already present. And if we are to believe some cell division theories, the disease has already been present for several years when the tumour is finally discovered. According to these theories, a visible tumour with an 8cm section needs 8 years to develop if the duplication period is 100 days. Every tumour starts with only one degenerate cell. If we assume duplication takes 100 days, a cell does need a considerable amount of time to grow into a visible tumour. Nevertheless, we are confronted with uncontrolled growth more and more nowadays, which makes a tumour even more serious.

We are faced with a nearly insoluble problem here. How can we detect a disease that is invisible and painless and of which the patient is unaware? We may pay a lot of attention to the early detection of tumours, but that is only possible up to a certain level. A cancer patient never shows specific symptoms. Nothing indicates the presence of cancer, until a tumour develops and starts pressing against an organ. After several years of experience with cancer patients, I have been able to determine a number of typical features, but they are not decisive enough to confirm the presence of cancer. That is why these typical features must never be generalized.

- Cancer patients have never or seldom been ill before.
- They seldom suffer from infectious illnesses.
- They seldom develop a fever.
- They never have ulcers.
- They never transpire heavily.
- They often have poor blood circulation.

- They do not care for sweet things.
- They eat very little fruit (very small amounts).
- They prefer things that taste salty.
- They do not have regular bowel movements.
- They are rather slim (not overweight).
- They often have an introverted character.
- They have trouble dealing with setbacks.

Some non-cancer patients also display these typical features; but it is noteworthy that cancer patients display a large number of them. People often ask me how they can distinguish a truly healthy person from a potential cancer patient, since neither is ever ill. As a generality, someone who is susceptible to cancer has a different aura, displays apathy or a kind of dullness. Nevertheless it still remains difficult to express assumptions merely in view of these typical features. It is not my intention to spread carcinophobia by publishing this list of features; on the contrary. I have often met people who possessed some of the features mentioned here. By acting on some good advice, they were able to get rid of those features. What also strikes me is that cancer patients who follow the Dries diet suddenly do start to transpire, develop a fever, get the flu and start to react to germs like any other person. Could that mean the recovery process has set in?

Oncology is not really concerned with studying the features of cancer patients. There is psychological research but most of the time the aim is to discover the psychological condition of the patient when the disease breaks out, how the patient reacts to the disease, or how he or she behaves during the course of the disease. Like any other science, medical science just happens to be characterized by a materialistic, analytical and technical aspect. This means that all research is based on studying matter, in this case the festering cells. When a biopsy is performed, the tissue is studied under a microscope and compared to healthy tissue. By 'analytical' I mean that medical science pays great attention to quantities. When a sample is taken, a check is made to see whether there are any cancer cells in the sample, or analysis is done of the composition of the blood or of the bodily fluids. The technical aspect has to do with the way in which the disease is treated: for cancer, that means surgery, chemotherapy or radiation. This all results in cancer being reduced to a medical–technical affair. Not everyone is satisfied with that. The treatment of cancer is always extremely aggressive and the side-effects are often worse than the disease itself, and all this while the results remain uncertain. Every oncologist is aware of this, but cancer just happens to be so aggressive that these treatments are nearly always necessary.

An Alternative Approach

It is necessary to turn to alternative treatments. Because oncology aims at saving human lives, it has no other choice but to accept regular treatments. But now a lot of people say: 'Everyone wants to live as long as possible, but not at just any price. Life has to remain bearable.' That is why additional or complementary therapies are also important. My diet, which I will describe later, is one of those complementary therapies. But before discussing that topic, I would like to have a look at another approach to cancer.

The material approach to cancer, as we know it from oncology, has its benefit and nobody doubts that, but we will never discover an adequate solution by looking at such a complex disease merely from a materialistic point of view. There are a number of indications that tell us we should interpret cancer in a different way. First of all, cancer is not a modern disease. The name *cancer* has existed for over 2,000 years and was first used by a Roman physician who compared an open breast cancer to a crayfish that had buried its legs in the surrounding tissue never to let go. *Kanker*, *cancer* and *krebs* are words that derived from the image of a crayfish: the crayfish is often used to symbolize cancer.

Nobody knows when cancer was first diagnosed, but we may

assume that it is quite an old disease, just like diabetes or rheumatism. These last two are described on the clay tablets of the ancient Babylonians, one of the oldest civilizations in the world. Even old Chinese writings accurately describe numerous diseases. It is most likely that cancer already existed in those days, but because of its insidious nature, it was only discovered later, in the Roman era. In the middle ages, all attention was focused on the plague, a disease caused by malnutrition and lack of hygiene. Even shortly before and during World War II, many people died of diseases that were never diagnosed. There is no doubt that one of those diseases was cancer. Even though cancer is a relatively old disease, it only became significant in the second half of the nineteenth century. During the industrial revolution, the number of cancer patients increased rapidly. Every time an agricultural society turned into an industrial society, the same thing happened. The strong industrial development of Western Europe, the USA and Japan was paralleled by an increased awareness of cancer, which undeniably has something to do with the way people live. An industrialized society is characterized by many factors that promote or cause cancer. Just think of the numerous chemicals, environmental pollution, the pollution of water supplies, heavy metals in the soil, certain additives in food, agricultural chemicals, increased radioactivity, etc. People who live in the Ruhr area of Germany are more susceptible to cancer than those who live on the Lüneburg Heath. The degree of civilization determines the degree of environmental pollution and therefore also the extent of the cancer risk. We have to distinguish cancer with an endogenous origin from cancer with an exogenous origin. Cancers that develop from the inside (out) belong to the first group (spontaneous cancers). Cancers caused by radioactive contamination, inhalation of asbestos fibres, chemicals, nicotine, etc. belong to the second group. For this last group, external factors are extremely important.

From the theoretical point of view, everyone is subjected to the same stimuli, yet one person develops cancer and another one does not. We have to distinguish being susceptible to cancer (individual problem), and cancer as a disease of mankind (common problem). Medical science mainly considers cancer an individual problem. Being susceptible obviously has to do with a number of individual characteristics (cancer resistance), which we will discuss later on. But it is a lot more important to find out how cancer developed as a disease of mankind.

Only man and his pets suffer from cancer. Wild animals do not get cancer, unless it is caused by serious environmental pollution. After the nuclear disaster in Chernobyl, insects were examined and young insects displayed a lot of defects. Therefore it is not inconceivable that increased radioactivity also causes cancer in animals. Under normal circumstances, animals that do not live in symbiosis with man do not get cancer. Cancer is considered a disease of civilization and is closely linked to our way of life.

The human is proud of being civilized. We think it is only natural that we live in concrete buildings; that water comes out of a tap; that we own a television set; that we wear clothes, travel by car, go to work, communicate by phone, take an aeroplane to go on a holiday, etc. Some even consider it unjust that a large part of the world's population does not have all this: providers of development aid to third world countries want to export a part of our civilization to them. But should we not ask ourselves this question: 'Is it normal that we live like this?' Should we not ask ourselves what price we have to pay in order to live the way we do? Everyone knows by now that our current industrial society has exceeded all standards and has reached its developmental limits. That is why we are trying to do something about the effects of industrialization, assuming our economical interests are not at risk though. We have to consider our current society as a scaled-up version of a much older society that was also wrong and in which cancer also existed. In the chaos of our larger, current society there is a proportional increase in the size of the problem, meaning we should look for the deeper cause elsewhere.

Ramapithecus is often seen as a distant ancestor of the modern human. It walked upright, lived on the plains and ate everything that was edible. It took a long time for Ramapithecus to evolve

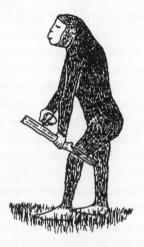

Figure 2 *Drawing of a Ramapithecus*

into *Homo sapiens*: this evolving humanity became more flawed the further it left the natural state behind. Because the laws of nature were taken into account less and less, the human became more susceptible to diseases. The human is the only creature on earth that suffers from so many diseases.

If we take look at the evolution of the human, we will notice that our ancestors are the same as those of the primates (tailless monkeys). Throughout that evolution, the human has managed to differentiate its behaviour from that of the primates. We do not know much about that distant past, except that the human has always been a frugivore – that is, a fruit-eater by nature. The famous paleologist Richard E Leakey has proven that beyond a doubt. Why else does the digestive system of the modern human – if we study its anatomy and physiology – still resemble that of a chimpanzee? There have been hardly any mutations.

Paleologists are mainly interested in the evolution of the man who walked upright and who was preceded by Ramapithecus. Paleologists and anthropologists are mainly interested in the cultural development of humankind, which explains their great interest in cranial capacity: the development of the brain made it more and more possible for the human to generate its own activities. The reader will probably not immediately notice a connection between cancer and the evolution of humankind; suffice it to say that what is decisive for the development of cancer in the human is civilization. At a certain point in evolution, the human decided to go its own way and tore itself away from the natural life; and that proved fatal to the human.

In spite of its cultural development, the human is still a natural creature, which means it is subjected to the laws of nature no matter what. But the human no longer allows itself to be guided by inner wisdom received from nature, putting faith instead in its own development and calling itself an autonomous creature. That leads to all kinds of problems for which the human itself finds solutions. Those solutions are not real though: they only have a temporary character. By fighting one disease, we create new diseases. Unfortunately I cannot explain these theories of natural philosophy any further, but I do want to point out that the deeper cause of cancer should be sought in that direction. We cannot develop an efficient method to fight cancer if we cannot gain a clear understanding of the correct cause of it. Because in this book I would like to limit myself to the practical aspect of this subject, I refer to the well-known saying: 'The history of disease is the history of agriculture.' This saying clearly illustrates that culture is unhealthy. Historical research has proved that all ancient civilizations had to deal with a large number of diseases. The Greek historians described the old Egyptians – with their fascinating and highly developed civilization – as a very unhealthy people. Egyptian medicine was quite well developed. Apart from that the Egyptians were very hygienic, which was not so much a luxury as a necessity. In almost all civilizations people pursued the independence of humankind from nature. In the course of its cultural history, humankind did everything to exceed the laws of nature as much as possible. In short, humans never took the laws of nature into account. Nevertheless our human body, or rather our whole human existence, depends on the laws of nature. Humankind and nature are indissolubly connected. If that bond is broken, humans become susceptible to diseases; the ills of our society confirm that.

In their wanderings throughout the plains, primitive humans ate everything that was somewhat edible, and spent a great deal of their time gathering food. Later they started hunting and fishing too. Only when grains and seeds of grasses were discovered did they succeed in preserving food for a longer period of time. The next step was to sow and harvest the grains and that was the birth of agriculture. The use of grains not only led to processing and preparation techniques but also to the use of sugar, salt and alcohol.

Practising agriculture and breeding stock forced humans to settle permanently, ending their nomadic life. Because of sufficient free time, they had the opportunity not only to develop new creative activities, but also to develop power politics. Archeological research shows that many ancient civilizations – like that of Central America (Incas and Mayas) – disappeared because of ecological disasters caused by their own development. Humans are extremely proud of their accomplishments but they are digging their own graves. Moreover they do not learn lessons from their own past. That is exactly why history keeps on repeating itself. The turns of the spiral become bigger and bigger. I can imagine these theories of natural philosophy seeming strange to some readers. But after reading this book they will agree that civilization is unhealthy. It is a well-known fact that civilizations unfamiliar with agriculture do not suffer from cancer, MS or other diseases of civilization. Is there no way for us to go back, even if we wanted to? In that respect the human is like a canary, imprisoned in its own system. A canary cannot be freed because it has been torn away from its natural environment, and stands no chance of surviving in nature. The system that imprisons humans is a fertile culture medium for all kinds of diseases. If we want to push back cancer, which is definitely desirable, we will have to make serious efforts to restore the damage to the environment, to provide healthy food, to create a better way of life and to adapt our economy. That does not only go for cancer but also for other diseases.

Proceeding from my belief in natural philosophy, I started looking for the right kind of food for humans. It did not take long for me to discover that agricultural products are actually not suitable for the human. If a cancer patient is fed as naturally as possible for three months – that is, without making use of agricultural products, without preparing the food (raw food) – his or her condition will certainly improve. After all the Dries diet is a fruit diet. It helps cancer patients switch back to their original food, the food their digestive system is made for. To recover from their illness, cancer patients need to go back to nature, which is logical since the disease is a consequence of an unnatural way of life. I do not wish to claim that you can get cancer by eating agricultural products, but on the other hand I am convinced that the human creature has become more susceptible to cancer and many other diseases because of having replaced original eating patterns by an artificial eating pattern. As I mentioned earlier, only humans and the animals they have domesticated suffer from cancer.

A few years ago, this point of view was still utopian, but now everything has changed. These last few years, many publications have mentioned the importance of phytochemicals. Phytochemicals are substances that are found in vegetarian food and that have a restraining influence on cancer. At the moment, every researcher, every cancer specialist is convinced of the fact that the polluted environment, disrupted society and industrialized food are the most important causes of cancer. Anyway there is enough evidence to prove it. That is why we can no longer limit ourselves to surgery, chemotherapy and radiation. We need complementary treatments that will improve the chances of recovery and that will reduce the side-effects. The best campaign against cancer is not to raise funds but to make people aware of the fact that our unnatural way of life (that is already thousands of years old) is the cause of this horrible disease. The progress of technology also adds to the problems.

Depending on the damage to the environment, 20–35 per cent of the population is affected by cancer.

Now that we know the deeper cause of cancer, it is a lot easier to fight it and to treat it. A disease such as cancer is more than just a physical problem that makes medical treatment necessary. Even more than other diseases, cancer makes us aware of the fact that we have to revolutionize our lives in order to conquer the disease. Cancer patients ask a lot of questions about the meaning of life, the coherence of things and the bond with nature. They have a great need for in-depth discussions. That is why it is not surprising that they ask us to pay attention to the psychological, the emotional and the social consequences of cancer.

A total approach of humans and their relationship with nature is extremely important. If cancer develops, a lot of things have to be done in a short period of time, and that is not always easy. When cancer strikes we are driven by a survival instinct that cannot always be separated from panic. We have to take so many important decisions that we can barely concentrate on complementary possibilities. Or else we do not even know they exist. As long as we only see the tumour and the possible consequences it may have, we 'feed' the disease and especially the panic it causes. We have to learn to think of life as it is and not as it is always presented to us. I have met some cancer patients who had the privilege of being familiar with this way of thinking: they managed to conquer their disease in nearly no time. The recovery process starts when you learn how to think in a different way. Those who are flexible enough to reorient themselves have a good chance of recovery, because they make themselves susceptible to the healing powers of nature that can mostly be found in food.

Cancer is not just a disease. It is a disease that is embedded in our society. All of us are denaturalized in such a way that we have created the disease ourselves. Because a number of unfortunate circumstances – often individually determined – come together some people develop cancer and others do not (yet). If we want to conquer cancer, we have no other choice but to return to nature, so that the unwell body can recover. This possibility offers new hope.

In natural medicine, illness is considered an attempt to recover. Disease has to do with life and not with death. Whoever becomes ill is offered a chance to repair his or her health. Cancer works in the same way other diseases do, but it does not have a language, or maybe we do not understand it!

Chapter 2

When Cancer Strikes

No one knows whether or not he is a carrier of the seeds of this horrible disease. Everyone can get cancer, which explains the continuous worry that often develops into carcinophobia or obsession. Sensible people opt for precautionary examination, since such examination has turned out to be very efficient for the early detection of breast cancer, uterine cancer and cervical cancer. Many women owe their lives to routine examination. Apart from that, routine examinations offer a certain kind of reassurance. For men, prostate examination can be very useful, because it makes the detection of a precancerous stage possible. Lung examination makes the early detection of lung cancer possible. But for most other cancers, precautionary examination proves to be rather difficult. Cancer prevention should not be restricted to medical examinations. It should also involve a healthy diet and a healthy way of life. If you follow a healthy diet and try to live in a healthy way, you are less likely to get cancer; and if cancer strikes anyway, you are more likely to recover from it.

We have to consider the fact that we are all at risk. But those that will not be counselled cannot be helped. Our environment has been damaged seriously: ambient radioactivity has increased; in some areas the soil is severely polluted and forests suffer from acid rainfall; high-voltage cables dangle above residential areas; and radiation from radar installations, broadcasting stations and satellites fills the air. Chemical and electromagnetic pollution are both serious in spite of a variety of measures taken to deal with them. Houses are often built with materials that either consist of or are treated with toxic substances. The food we eat and the drinks we consume are polluted because they contain so many additives. Bad habits – such as drinking alcohol or smoking – do damage our health, even though Dr De Veer, biochemist and author of several health books, says that 90 per cent of heavy smokers do not develop cancer. That is cold comfort though. Our way of life has become a complete chaos: aggressive advertising forces us to buy all kinds of useless things; the media provide us with so much information that we can barely deal with it; silence has been replaced by noise and commercial music; education is becoming increasingly demanding; and professional life has lost every form of creativity. Modern humanity is burdened with the problems of a consumer society. Because we are denaturalized, we are becoming more susceptible to diseases such as cancer every day. Everyone is alarmed by the growing number of cancer cases. But we must not lose control, in spite of everything, and not let every little lump or bump, every persistent cough or continuous hoarseness confuse us. We must not worry too much or start searching our bodies for something suspicious every day. That would make life quite intolerable.

A distinction has to be made between the general fear of being struck by cancer and the state of actually having cancer. When something abnormal is discovered or suspected, we must keep calm and consult a GP without delay. Very often women have already had a lump in their breast for months before they finally consult their GP. The thought that they might have cancer alarms them, but they forget that living in uncertainty is also unbearable. Denial may be a temporary solution, but it may have a fatal ending as well. A suspicion always has to be confirmed or denied. I have often seen people who were really terrified. But once they knew they had cancer, their fear disappeared and made way for courage. I have also seen several people die because they did not have the courage to consult their GP. And although they were prepared to follow nutritional therapy, it turned out to be an impossible option because cancer had already overwhelmed them. They had waited too long.

Because research is done by various specialists in various laboratories, it may take weeks before a final verdict can be decided. For some people it is very difficult to wait over that period of time. It is certainly not easy to live between hope and despair. One moment they believe in false alarm, and the next moment they are firmly convinced the worst awaits them. Then there are the sleepless nights, the hopeless pessimism, the lack of appetite resulting in severe weight loss, the horrible times at which one breaks out in tears while another bottles everything up and wants to talk to no one. And even when the test results are positive the emotional or psychological wounds are deep. People should not be kept in suspense for so long, waiting for a diagnosis. Relatives of cancer patients live with the continuous fear that they themselves might develop cancer sooner or later, knowing that cancer is not hereditary but that hereditary defects, such as an increased chance of cancer, do exist. The only defence we have against cancer is to stay calm, feel healthy and live as normally as possible. Fear is our greatest enemy. Fear can destroy entire lives.

In a recent brochure the Flemish Cancer League stated that 'medical terminology is far too complicated, too vague, too obscure for many. Whoever is worried has the right to a serious and competent judgement. Unnecessary worry can only be prevented by providing clear, explicit and comprehensible information. And even that is no guarantee, because someone who is really scared of cancer – and who isn't? – may not hear the whole story and only remember fragments of what has been said.' Organizations (such as those listed at the back of this book), information services and even good literature can be helpful sources of information, but eventually the patient expects a clear answer from a physician. Only the answer of a physician provides absolute certainty.

An open conversation with relatives, friends or acquaintances can offer great relief, even though those people cannot offer you certainty. It is important for cancer patients to express themselves, to find a release and to be able to share their sorrow. Men generally find that extremely difficult. Society teaches men to be strong, to not cry. They often adopt a businesslike attitude towards the outside world, while deep in their hearts they are begging for comfort. There are some fortunate men who are not afraid to ask their wives for comfort and understanding, because even that is something many men cannot manage to do.

When cancer strikes it is obvious that the GP should be the first person to be consulted. Even though a GP is consulted by cancer patients regularly, dealing with cancer remains difficult for both parties. Patients often suspect a GP is not qualified enough to deal with cancer, even though they know better. The GP's job is not easy either: on one hand he or she must not cause the patient to panic needlessly, and on the other hand he or she must not seem indifferent. Many patients are very demanding, and seek the impossible from their GPs. Usually it is the GP who refers the patient to a medical specialist or who arranges hospitalization.

Just like the patient, the GP has to wait for the final results. In fact the GP has to deal with the same uncertainty. Not every GP is capable of setting aside his or her strictly medical pattern of thought to have an informal chat. A GP often lacks the time to do so. But once the patient has been diagnosed and the treatment has been taken over by a specialist, the function of the GP changes completely, which improves the relationship between the GP and the cancer patient. A lot of cancer patients speak highly of the good relationship between themselves and their GPs. Specialists and cancer patients seldom develop a close relationship because there is too much distance between them. The large hospital, the medical equipment, the variety of specialists, the growing medical record and the routine treatments offer little warmth, little opportunity for deeply human contact. Nevertheless it does happen more and more often that a specialist really sympathizes with his or her patient and develops a less formal relationship with him or her.

Nevertheless, a specialist is often stuck in a system with its daily routine. The patient is often overwhelmed by the many strange impressions of the large hospital and is often not capable of asking questions. The patient is not prepared for what is happening to him or her and, moreover, it all happens extremely fast. People should be more informed, more aware of what is going on. They should ask more questions. A patient has the right to know what he or she is suffering from and how serious the illness is. He or she has to know about the method(s) of treatment and what risks the treatment involves. There are people who trust medical science implicitly. If all ends well there is no problem, but if there are complications or if the outcome is fatal, there is a lot of criticism. All this makes people very distrustful of medicine and that should be avoided. One cancer patient who was very familiar with medical treatments told me that most cancer patients know very little about both regular and complementary treatments.

It is important for cancer patients to receive support during the first stage of their illness. They especially need care when they are still in the stage in which they strongly suspect they have cancer. I have often been contacted by people who had been through a preliminary examination. The mere fact that these people were able to talk about their problems not only gave them relief but also strength. When I told them about the possibilities and most of all the advantages of nutritional therapy, it gave them a little bit of certainty. Those who opened their minds to nutritional therapy were all in a privileged position anyhow, as they were advantaged by their general mental outlook.

Unfortunately I have also met people whose story was so worrying that I did not have to wait for the diagnosis; I knew the outcome would be fatal. It is much more difficult to find words of comfort and strength for people like that. They look at you as if you do not want to help them, when in fact they demand the impossible. In such cases we wait for the diagnosis and the prognosis and then we usually suggest palliative care, in which a special diet can also play a part.

The Naked Truth

After weeks of fear and uncertainty the patient is suddenly told: 'We have some bad news, it is indeed malignant.' This subtle and well-wrapped announcement is a heavy blow. The patient often comforts him- or herself with the words 'I thought so'. It is impossible to determine what goes through the patient's mind at that moment. It is like a stroke of lightning. It seems as if the patient's blood curdles, as if his or her breath is cut off. His or her whole future collapses like a house of cards. Everyone reacts in his or her own way, though. Some seem stunned or completely indifferent, and barely know what has been said. Others become rebellious or aggressive, and fly into a temper. Still others are courageous and are determined to recover at any cost.

Some physicians are quite good at disguising the announcement without bending the truth. They inform the patient of the therapeutic possibilities and the realistic chance of survival. Other physicians are impersonal and brief when they talk to a patient. Once the patient is informed, they close the file and stand up, which means: 'You may leave now'. What is routine for the physician is like a death sentence for the patient, though, even if the prognosis is positive.

Some physicians are extremely callous. Maybe having to deal with death daily makes people that way. One cancer patient told me he suffered from a cold that would not go away. That worried him, so he consulted his GP. His GP suspected more and referred him to the hospital for further examination. A few weeks later he was invited to see a specialist. The specialist opened his file and immediately told him he suffered from a severe form of cancer. 'Why don't you go home and take care of business because you don't have much time left?' he was told. Of course the patient was completely taken by surprise. There is certainly no point in giving false hope to someone with very little chance of survival, but on the other hand we must not forget that a person cannot live without hope. When making such an announcement, one should at least discuss how the illness ran its course. One should use words of comfort and strength. A physician should prepare him- or herself thoroughly to perform such a duty. He or she has to make sure the patient is accompanied by a trusted person when he or she comes to the health centre, for it is irresponsible to allow someone who has just received a life-threatening message to go home alone. One possibility is to make sure the patient is accompanied by someone such as a psychologist or a social worker. Another patient was also told the plain truth straight to his face. He drove home, killed his wife and then himself. This family crisis could have been avoided if the physician had prepared his or her announcement more carefully or if he or she had chosen other words.

It is obviously also a good idea for the patient to be accompanied by his or her partner or other trusted person. Sometimes a patient has to leave the clinic all by him- or herself. Completely dazed and crushed, he or she has to deal with his or her sorrow alone. Hospitals have become very industrialized in recent years. They have become real enterprises. Members of staff often bear more resemblance to robots than to trained nurses. That is not the fault of the personnel, nor is it the fault of the government that enforces economy measures. The whole situation is caused by the enormous need for medical care and a general lack of financial resources with which to meet the overwhelming demand. These days nearly everyone makes use of the health service and that is not how it was originally supposed to work. All this has led to mergers and over-sized hospitals.

Unfortunately small, friendly hospitals that are able to show a little warmth and affection no longer exist. And if there still were a hospital like that, the patient would not trust going there for various reasons: it might be felt that the equipment is outdated or that there is a lack of equipment or specialists. On the other hand it is also obvious that patients cannot feel at ease in a mega-hospital, which can seem characterized by alienation between physicians and patients. Many people are under the impression that hospitals treat them like children. A physician does not speak the language of his or her patients, he or she only speaks the language of medical science, only sees the disease – in the case of cancer that means the tumour – and is barely interested in the person who carries the tumour. I am not claiming that it is always like that, but there are patients who are under that impression, especially because some physicians hardly make any effort to avoid that impression. In the eyes of the patient, the physician is the guardian angel who has to take care of everything, but in reality his or her job is rather limited. His or her duty is to remove the tumour surgically from the patient hidden under the green sheet. The only hole in the sheet is located wherever the surgery will be performed. Surgery is a technical operation that is performed by highly qualified medical practitioners. Any remaining and/or hidden cells are killed by means of chemotherapy or radiation treatment, which of course is the job of other specialists. The personal involvement of a specialist in the recovery process is minimal and is limited to only one of the many medical treatments. That is exactly what the multidisciplinary system is all about. There is no other way, since even a hospital is subjected to the laws of the economy.

Many people say: 'I hope I never end up in a hospital'. It is very likely that patients expect too much from hospitals or from physicians. Do we not all value our own lives very highly, especially when they are threatened? We often mistake the physician for a magician who can and will make our problems disappear. On one hand we criticize medicine but on the other hand we all feel we depend on it. One female patient was so disappointed about the care and attention she received in a large clinic that she refused medical aid for a long time. 'They are all murderers', she yelled. Every time she went to the hospital, she saw a different specialist, someone who did not even know her medical history. The professor who had operated on her never had time for her, and always sent an assistant. I know the professor probably had something more important to do than to check on a post-operative patient, which can be done just as well by an assistant. But in the eyes of the patient it seemed as if he did not have time for her while he did for others.

A hospital is still considered a life-saving institution while it is in fact a place where a lot of people die. We have to realize that this world is being destroyed by its own complicated systems. It is idealistic to expect the hospital staff to welcome you with open arms, to expect they will always be able to spend sufficient time on your problems. You are just one of many, just as the physician is one of many physicians. A physician can only make a limited amount of time available for you, and even so only to deal with a medical aspect he or she is authorized for. In a five-star hotel you are also left to fend for yourself, even though there may be a rose on your pillow and a welcome card on the bedside table. That happens to be exactly what you paid for. If your washing machine breaks down, it is up to you to phone a mechanic. No one else will worry about the dirty laundry that cannot be washed. No one worries about the fact that a faulty washing machine is a complete disaster for a housewife. Our world is indifferent and there is nothing we can do about it, except to try to be a little more considerate.

To criticize medicine is in fact nothing other than to react to the wrongs of our society. Life in hospitals is no better or worse than anywhere else. In times of need, we are more susceptible to certain situations. If you are ever confronted with cancer it is a good idea to build up your self-confidence and determination. If you cannot do that yourself, allow someone to help you. The best thing you can do, though, is to take control of your own life and not expect too much from others.

It is very positive that people are being told the truth nowadays. In the past, many patients were told stories and only the relatives were informed of the seriousness of the disease. The word 'cancer' was not to be used, because its insensitive use could lead to unnecessary worrying by the patient. I still remember the times when I had to promote the cancer diet without using the word 'cancer'. I have seen people who had had to undergo chemotherapy and who had experienced hair loss, and still had not been told they had cancer. A long time ago there was a man in my waiting room who said to another patient: 'I have cancer, but they don't want to tell me.' This seldom happens these days. It must be horrible for a patient not being able to talk about his or her illness with his or her partner or children, knowing he or she cannot prepare his or her farewell. The moment the cancer is confirmed, he or she can at least start to offer resistance: from that moment on, he or she can actively participate in his or her recovery process. It is remarkable how extremely courageous cancer patients can be.

When in Doubt

Sometimes the diagnosis is very well described. That means the physician is able to determine the exact condition of the patient. He or she knows the exact size of the tumour; the tumour is well-enclosed and easily removable, without risk of metastasis; chemotherapy will only be used as a precautionary measure; the prognosis is favourable. In this case it will be easy for the patient to trust the surgeon. But sometimes the physician does not know exactly what is going on. Sometimes there are doubts: 'Is this the main tumour or a secondary tumour? Do we remove the uterus or not?' These doubts do not depend on the skill of the specialist but on the complexity of the disease. In these cases it is wise to consult a specialist of another hospital. You do not have to repeat all the examinations, but you can ask another specialist for a second opinion, since he or she may have a better proposition. I know one young woman who went to a gynaecologist to have her uterus examined. After an extensive examination the gynaecologist said: 'You'd better stay here. That way we can perform surgery tomorrow morning.' The woman, who was very alert and determined, immediately said: 'Never. I at least want to sleep on such an important decision.' She was in terror when she phoned me and asked me for advice. I told her to consult another gynaecologist for a second opinion, which she did. She did not have the operation and a year later she even gave birth to a healthy son. When one has cancer, one should neither waste time nor make rash decisions.

The Treatment

Cancer patients react in different ways. Some experience the tumour as a kind of devil they want to exorcize as soon as possible; others keep on postponing decisions. The fear of surgery is often deep-rooted. In the past it used to be said that exposing cancer to light increased the chance of metastasis; but that was before World War II, at a time when the treatment of cancer was still very inefficient. Patients who did not have their tumours removed were more likely to recover than those who underwent surgery and treatment. That was at the beginning of the biological fight against cancer. Now things are different. Surgery is performed under much more favourable circumstances, and always quite accurately. Some risks can never be avoided, though. A tumour is a time bomb that can explode at any time. Some tumours are not so dangerous. They are well enclosed and do not entail immediate danger. Other tumours grow rapidly and one never knows in which direction they will grow, with surgery absolutely necessary in most cases, unless the condition of the patient is so serious that there is no chance of survival. The disadvantages of surgery are generally known: impairment of the defence mechanism as a result of anaesthesia, traumatic shock, physical and psychological stress. There is always the possibility of the tumour emptying itself during surgery, causing the release of cancer cells. That possibility cannot always be eliminated. Nevertheless, these disadvantages are nothing compared to the danger a tumour involves. Some people are too scared to undergo surgery. I try to help them get over their fear by making them aware of the danger they are in. If they still wish to refuse surgery, I usually apply the Dries diet for a period of three months. We then wait for the tumour to shrivel, which unfortunately does not always happen: it may do so and it has done so in the past, but there is no guarantee. Every case is different, every person reacts in a different way. Several times I have found that tumours that *could not* be removed surgically at first (because the patient had waited too long) had shrivelled in such a way that they *could* be removed, and all this after application of the Dries diet. This has mostly happened with brain tumours that had not been, or had only partially been, removed because of their location. Very often the remaining tumour of a patient who had followed my diet disappeared completely. The question is: Why perform surgery if we can also do it this way? Postponing surgery can bring about certain risks, and taking risks is exactly what you should avoid when you have cancer.

One cancer patient who had had a prior operation asked me for advice. She had a new tumour, located near the left collarbone. She did not, however, want to go back to hospital where she had been treated before. The reason – she told me – was that a female physician had told her to abandon further examination and not have the tumour removed. 'After all, the tumour is well enclosed,' were her exact words. I can understand why people do not want to undergo surgery every other day, but to refuse examination seems irresponsible to me. The patient consulted me regularly and every time I could see that her insecurity had grown. Then I told her: 'If your physician is so sure the tumour is well enclosed, the chance of it releasing cancer cells is very minimal indeed.' But because her condition got worse and worse, she was finally forced to call in medical assistance. The examination indicated that two other tumours were hidden under the known tumour.

A few years ago, the general tendency was to perform breast-saving surgery. Now that decision has been reconsidered, especially because many tumours can reappear. During an ideal operation, the tumour is removed completely, but the disease is not: removing a symptom of a disease is not the same as eliminating its cause. An operation has to be seen as a means of limiting immediate danger as much as possible. Most cancer patients easily opt for an operation. With chemotherapy that is not the case.

Chemotherapy

Most people want to avoid chemotherapy at all costs, and ask their physician if it is really necessary. In recent years scientists have been able to develop a whole range of chemical treatments, but chemotherapy remains a serious and especially aggressive therapy. Cytostatics involves killing the cells from the outside, using highly toxic substances. Up to a few decades ago more people died of cytostatics than of cancer. Luckily, things have changed. Everyone wants to survive and knowingly take risks in order to survive. Most cancer patients recover quite well after an operation, but the results of chemotherapy are very different. Even people who normally look dazzling look like wrecks after their first treatment with chemotherapy. Hair loss and nausea still seem acceptable side-effects compared to the collapse of the defence mechanism and the damage caused to the gastro-intestinal tract. Patients who have enough strength to overcome the side-effects of the chemotherapy benefit from it. Unfortunately no one knows in advance who can and who cannot endure it. One of the main purposes of the Dries diet is to enable cancer patients to reduce the side-effects of chemotherapy as much as possible. A large number of my patients – especially those who started applying the Dries diet early – have succeeded in doing so quite well.

One of my patients was nicknamed 'the iron man' by the hospital staff because he came through the chemotherapy with flying colours. Other patients barely experienced hair loss, did not develop nausea and showed few traces of damage. The use of a herbal tea with strongly purifying and excretory effects clears the body in no time. This is explained mor elaborately in chapter 6, in which I discuss the practical applications of the diet. Applying chemotherapy can be compared to extinguishing a fire. When there is a fire, the fire brigade has to take action to prevent everything from burning down. After the fire has been extinguished there may, however, be more water damage than fire damage. The fight against cancer finds itself in the same delicate situation: you have to destroy everything in order to make the most of a nearly hopeless situation.

It remains very difficult for oncologists to draw up a balance sheet in advance. Sometimes cancer patients cannot handle the chemotherapy any more and therefore interrupt the treatment prematurely. In many cases it turns out that it was the right decision, especially when the cancer was already out of control anyway. The months or weeks that remained were spent in a bearable and – more importantly – a human way. Personally, I feel that a cancer patient should keep on fighting, since there is always a chance of sudden change, no matter how advanced the disease. Nevertheless there is a limit. And once that limit has been reached there is only one choice left. Palliative treatment is the best choice at that time.

All oncologists agree that chemotherapy is an aggressive therapy with a lot of disadvantages. They assume that high doses repeated shortly after each other are the most effective. But because of that procedure the patient does not have the opportunity to produce a sufficient number of white blood cells. It also means that the defence mechanism lacks time to recover and gets the whole works over and over again. If the chemotherapy could be spread over a longer period of time, the effects would not be so dramatic. The fact that the required dose of cytostatics is enormous shows how persistent cancer is. Patients who apply the Dries diet are more capable of building up their defence mechanisms, while waste products leave their bodies sooner.

People often ask me what it is like to fight cancer merely by applying a diet. In the past, certain cancer patients told me they were convinced that patients who applied a diet were in no need of chemotherapy or of radiation. But five years later they were completely consumed by cancer. In some cases the tumour had grown so much that surgery had become impossible. During the past few years there have been several important attempts to find an alternative solution, but I know that that day has not come yet. I know cancer patients who followed my diet and recovered completely, without needing an operation or chemotherapy, but others have died. Because we are not at liberty to take risks, I am in favour of applying regular treatments and complementing them with the diet. After all, it is this combination that produces the best results. Most people who try to fight cancer biologically make the mistake of shouting victory too soon, and of condemning regular medicine. Everything for them is seen from a black-and-white point of view.

I am absolutely certain that a large number of patients who apply my diet no longer have to undergo chemotherapy or radiation treatment. Some may be able to stop the treatments early or adjust the doses. Several times the oncologist has decided that the condition of the patient allowed him or her to discontinue the treatment early. But the decision whether or not to apply chemotherapy has to be made by both the patient and the oncologist. As a dietician I am not authorized to do that. If the positive results of the Dries diet continue to increase in number, we will deal with chemotherapy differently in the future. But one major condition has to be fulfilled: the patient has to apply the diet strictly for a certain period of time.

The Dries diet has made chemotherapy a lot more bearable. It limits the side-effects, it allows the defence mechanism to recover and it helps the body get rid of toxic substances more rapidly. To complement chemotherapy with the Dries diet is highly recommended. I believe that everyone should follow it. After all it is a decision which a patient can make on his or her own, a decision to which no oncologist would object.

Radiation Treatment

Radiation treatment or radiotherapy is also used to kill cancer cells. A primary, curative radiation treatment is applied in cases for which experience has taught us that radiotherapy has better results. Radiotherapy is often used in combination with chemotherapy. Palliative radiation treatment is mainly used to suppress pain, and cannot only lengthen life but also improve its quality.

There are different kinds of ray and different ways in which to apply radiation treatment; to determine the appropriate kind of such treatment, its dose and its duration, various factors have to be taken into account.

Just like chemotherapy, radiotherapy has a number of side-effects, both general and local. Some general side-effects are: fatigue, need for rest and sleep and decrease of appetite. These side-effects are caused by the toxic substances that are produced as a result of the decomposition of cells. Whether nausea and vomiting occur depends mostly on the size of the radiation field and the dose of radiation. Nausea and vomiting are more likely to occur when radiation treatment is applied to the abdominal organs. Nevertheless, these side-effects may also occur when the radiation treatment is applied to other parts of the body.

Local side-effects are in fact reactions to the radiation. They are caused by the normal tissue that is situated in the radiation field. Complaints of this nature disappear easily and within a short period of time. Patients who have to undergo radiation treatment of the skull suffer from hair loss. Sometimes the skin, the oesophagus, the intestines and the bone marrow are also damaged. For the entire duration of the radiation treatment, the number of leucocytes and thrombocytes is determined at least once a week. This procedure makes it possible to diagnose the damage to the bone marrow and the seriousness of that damage, so that the dose of radiation can be adapted if necessary. The number of times a patient can go through chemotherapy or radiation treatment is limited. Especially cancer patients who relapse will quickly reach the maximum number of treatments. After that the Dries diet is often the only possible therapy. And even in cases like that we have been able to produce positive results. The only condition has been that the diet had to be applied for a long period of time, usually a year.

Radiotherapy severely damages the defence system. By applying the Dries diet the side-effects are reduced and damage can be repaired more rapidly, at least to the extent that it *can* be repaired. That is certainly an enormous advantage.

If chemotherapy and/or radiation treatment do not have the expected results, patients are very disappointed, and they wish they had backed out of those aggressive methods. Whenever the patient dies, the relatives always agree that – should they be given a second chance – they would never opt for the same kind of treatment again. 'We shouldn't have done that to him or her,' may people think, while only blaming themselves. They seem to forget that you cannot force someone to go through radiotherapy or chemotherapy against his or her own will. Moreover, the patient always has the right to discontinue treatment; he or she has to make that decision. Sometimes that is extremely difficult, though, especially because the patient is confronted with a very tense situation and has no idea of his or her own condition; and, finally, because the decision has to be made quickly. A patient or a relative of a patient cannot assess the seriousness of the disease or the chance of survival. After all, that is the job of the physician. That is why such a decision is usually made by the physician. Patients ask: 'What would you do in my case?' The standard answer to that question is: 'Treat it as soon as possible.' When a disease is so far advanced that treatment is useless, that is exactly what the physician will tell his or her patient. When on the other hand the physician decides to apply a treatment, it is because he or she hopes it is the right decision (just as his or her patient does). It means that both the physician and the patient think there is a chance of recovery. The problem is that there is no alternative. You cannot treat cancer with beetroot juice or sauerkraut. It would seem that people who discontinue their treatment because they cannot bear it any more, easily lose confidence in the medical staff attending them, because afterwards they often say: 'When we stopped the treatment, the whole hospital staff turned against us'.

A patient must not take serious decisions in a few minutes and certainly not during a first conversation, but should sleep on the decision and discuss his or her decision with relatives first. Even though chemotherapy and radiotherapy are horrible experiences, everyone hopes they can be saved by these aggressive methods.

Someone who rejects treatment usually feels he or she has given up, a feeling followed by this thought: 'There is nothing to be done anyway.' If there is really nothing to be done, these therapies are pointless indeed, and only make the patient more ill than he or she already is. I once visited a colleague in hospital, and he said: 'I have discussed all the possibilities with the physician. I do not stand a chance, which is why I have chosen palliative care.' I was taken by surprise by his decision, because he was only 42 years old. Later, it seemed he had made the right choice. Up to four months before his death he still went jogging weekly, I saw him at a meeting, and he kept in touch. It still happens regularly that cancer is only discovered in such a late stage.

The largest group of cancer patients falls between the group of those whose cancer is discovered early and that of those who are terminal cases. This means that those in the large middle group have to deal with great uncertainty. They cannot give up on everything at this stage: after all there is still a chance of recovery. Because most cancer patients belong to this middle group, they mainly tend to agree to the proposed treatment.

Most people do not realize that chemotherapy and radio-therapy are merely attempts to kill the present or possibly present cancer cells. No individual oncologist can offer absolute certainty. Every cancer patient reacts in a different way; every cancer patient is different. One patient, who – together with his family – had started applying a healthy diet six years earlier, was suddenly confronted with intestinal cancer. The examination showed there was an 8cm tumour at the end of the large intestine. The patient had already consulted me prior to the operation and immediately started with the Dries diet. The surgeon was stupefied when he saw the man recover completely in just a few days time, after such a serious and long operation. 'Other patients need two weeks or more to do that,' he told his patient. The oncologist who discussed the proposed treatment with the patient decided to apply neither chemotherapy nor radiotherapy. He made a realistic statement: 'Chemotherapy does not offer more certainty than the diet you are applying right now.' I agree completely with that statement. Furthermore, I am pleased to note that people who have not had chemotherapy or radiotherapy react extremely well to my diet. The man I told you about earlier still goes for check-ups regularly and his condition is improving remarkably well. The six years of healthy diet were definitely a foundation for him to build on. Meanwhile I am convinced that prevention is about adapting your diet and lifestyle in such a way that – if cancer strikes – you are more likely to recover, so that chemotherapy and radiotherapy may not be needed.

Every recovery process is nourished by hope. Opting for chemotherapy or radiotherapy can be part of that hope, just like refusing it because of fear or despair. If a patient chooses to receive aggressive treatments, he or she has to realize that complementary diets and other complementary therapies are an absolute must. Dr R De Greef says: 'Patients often turn to alternative therapies hoping they can avoid the regular therapies. If the regular therapies prove to be necessary, they drop the alternative therapies, while it is exactly at that time that they can be most helpful.'[1] People still think that they have to choose between regular or alternative treatments, but it is not a choice they have to make: the best thing to do is to choose a suitable regular treatment and a complementary treatment to go with it (just as the term 'complementary' suggests).

Sometimes hospitalization is an inevitable choice, especially when medical treatment or pain treatment is necessary. Naturally home care is ideal, but unfortunately it is not always feasible. It is not easy to adjust to a situation that sometimes changes from day to day. I have known many terminal patients who were sent home without any form of treatment. Of course they had to go to the hospital for check-ups regularly, but that was nothing more than a psychological compensation. Because they did not want to acknowledge their hopeless situation or

[1] Dr R De Greef, *Immunologie*, Arinus, Genk, 1992, p. 34.

because they were counting on delay, they immediately started to apply the Dries diet. In most cases the hospital staff was surprised about the fact that these patients remained 'well' for so long, without needing medical attention. Several patients were even thought to go through a sudden change of condition at a certain point. In any case, every one of them was able to lengthen his or her life and improve its quality, while barely needing – or even without needing – medical treatment, because there was no pain or discomfort. That is one good reason for applying the Dries diet.

Chapter 3

The Bio-energetic Aspect

In the first chapter I discussed the insidious nature of cancer and I mentioned that medical science is based on materialistic principles – that is, on tangible research. Medical science studies mainly visible data; that is why medical science speaks of cancer only when there is a clearly perceptible tumour. Oncology tells us that a visible tumour is the result of at least 25 multiplications of the cells. If we assume duplication takes place every 100 days, we can compute how many years go by before we can detect a tumour. From the aetiological point of view the cancer has already been there for all those years. Cancer is a disease that causes a cell to mutate and makes it possible for one degenerate cell to develop into a tumour. That latent aspect of cancer is exactly what makes the disease so terrifying. It certainly makes sense to study visible tumours, to help us gain insight into the way they originate, develop and spread. But the invisible or bio-energetic aspect is equally important. Bio-energetic research opens new perspectives and most of all gives new hope. I will not discuss it in detail here, but I do think it necessary to give a brief description that will not only clarify the link between bio-energy and cancer but also the link between bio-energy and food. After all, my diet is based on bio-energy.

It was in 1924 that Russian scientist Alexander Gurwitsch carried out his famous onion experiment which proved that plants are capable of storing and radiating light energy. For his

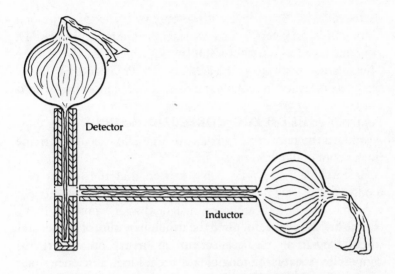

Figure 3 *Gurwitsch's onion experiment (according to Popp)*
If you join the roots of the two onions you will notice that one influences the
other, since the cell division in both roots increases

experiment he used transparent and opaque glass plates, which
he placed between the roots of two onions. When he used the
transparent glass plates, he was able to determine the influence of
the roots of one onion on the roots of the other onion. When he
used the opaque glass plates, nothing happened. That made
Gurwitsch conclude that there was an emission of light energy.
He was convinced his theory would change the world of science
profoundly, because it added a non-material aspect to the
material aspect.

Even though the Gurwitsch experiment is mentioned in many
books, nobody has ever really paid any attention to it, mainly
because it was not possible to investigate such experiments accurately in those days; moreover, the times were not yet ripe for that.
In the 1950s, an Italian team repeated Gurwitsch's experiment,
because better and more accurate measuring instruments were by

then available. Nevertheless it was only in 1974 – 50 years after Gurwitsch's discovery – that the famous German physicist Dr Popp managed to carry out a similar experiment. In 1982, at the Max Planck Institute of Heidelberg, Dr Popp and his fellow workers succeeded in proving the presence of biophotons or units of light in vegetable organisms. One of the fellow workers of Dr Popp proved that those biophotons are stored in DNA. Dr Popp developed the measuring instruments that allow us to determine the amount of biophotons in a foodstuff.

Research led by Dr Popp has proven that the quality of a foodstuff is mainly determined by the amount of biophotons it contains. Biophotons are units of light that are found in living organisms, as opposed to photons, which may also be found elsewhere. Upgrading and chemical cultivation of foodstuffs are true dangers to the biophotons as are processing, conserving and storing of foodstuffs. What Dr Popp has discovered in his laboratory only very recently, had already been put into practice by (among others) Dr Nolfi, who was the first to use raw food in the fight against cancer. In my book *Natural Food for Daily Use* (1977), I wrote that food should not be industrially processed and that we had no other choice but to return to pure, natural food, which explains the title.

Dr Popp assumes that the human and other animals are not calorie-eaters but absorbers of light. During photosynthesis a plant absorbs sunlight and converts it into chemical energy; carbon dioxide and water are converted into dextrose. Animals and humans – who live on plants, either directly or indirectly – decompose those sugar molecules, turning them into carbon dioxide and water once again. The total amount of carbon dioxide an animal or a human produces is expelled by the lungs and breathed out. The water leaves the human body through skin (perspiration), urine and bowel movement. A part of the solar energy that plants absorb and that is not used for photosynthesis is stored in their DNA. When we eat plants, that sublimed solar energy ends up in our bodies, where it helps our entire organisms function in a way we cannot yet explain.

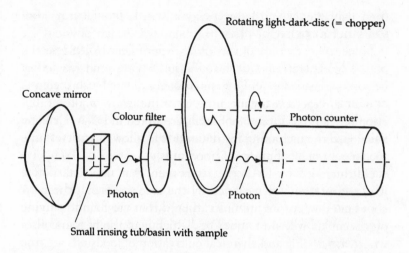

Figure 4 *Principle used to measure the amount of biophotons, according to Prof. Dr Popp*

Dr Popp has proven in a scientific way that the quality of a foodstuff depends on its ability to store and retain light energy. According to him, not only the nutritional value but also the healing power of a foodstuff depends on the amount of light energy that is retained in the plant. If the amount of light energy in a fresh leaf is measured, a very high value can be determined, while a withered leaf of the same plant will indicate barely any value. When the luminous intensity of both leaves is displayed on a screen, it can be seen that the fresh leaf has a very powerful luminous intensity, while the withered leaf's luminous intensity is strongly reduced. Dr Popp's research can be called revolutionary. It gives a whole new meaning to observation of food, health and illness.

Dr Popp's research is based on quantitative measurements of biophotons in foodstuffs. From that we may conclude the following: the more biophotons there are in a foodstuff, the higher the quality of that foodstuff. Humans and other animals need light energy and light energy is mainly provided by food-stuffs that are rich in biophotons.

Since the beginning of the 1980s, I have been doing research on the bio-energetic value of foodstuffs. My research should not be confused with that of Dr Popp, though, even though there is a close link. Not only the amount of biophotons is important, but also the luminous intensity of the light energy. The bio-energetic value (BEV) of a foodstuff is determined by the intensity of one biophoton, since all photons have an equal intensity. To understand this, we have to understand a number of concepts. Those who are interested in further explanation can consult the book about bio-energy I mentioned earlier. But in view of the purpose of this book, I will limit myself to discussing the main principle of bio-energy.

The scientific study of energy tells us that energy moves at the speed of light and by means of waves. A wave has a certain length, which is called a wavelength. A wavelength can be very long, which means it stretches over several kilometres, but it can also be very short (so-called microwaves).

Wavelength is proportionate to frequency. Frequency means the number of cycles per second. If the wave is short, the frequency is high and if the wave is long, the frequency is low, because the speed of light is an invariable.

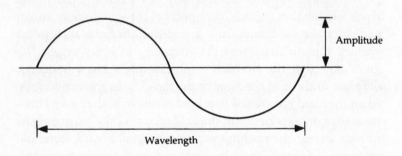

Figure 5 *Wavelength and amplitude*

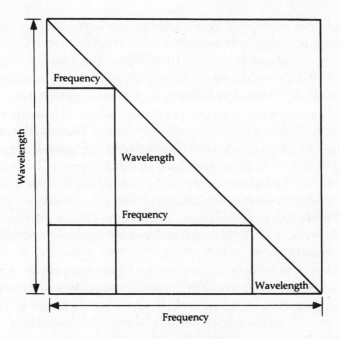

Figure 6 *Frequency diagram*

The bio-energetic value of a foodstuff is measured by means of a Lecher antenna, a very accurate measuring instrument developed by the German engineer Schneider, who based his work on the parallel system of the German Prof. Dr Lecher. Students of physics know that there is a connection between human energy and microwaves. Schneider's knowledge of space technology enabled him to determine the frequency of every organ. We know now that the stomach – for example – has a frequency different to those of the liver or the muscles. In the early 1980s, when they had just started that kind of research, they asked me – because of my experience in the field of nutrition – to investigate to what extent the readings were meaningful. Soon I found out that each foodstuff could be identified by a certain frequency, since they all had different frequencies. A high reading means a high bio-energetic value. Popular medicine and my own experience indicate that certain foodstuffs can be used to support a certain organ, or to cure a certain disease. We wanted to know whether this could also be verified by means of bio-energetic readings. We were extremely surprised when we discovered that the readings allowed us to determine the medicinal properties of both foodstuffs and herbs very accurately. Based on this experience I started to develop diets for several illnesses. That was also my motive for developing a cancer diet.

When I started publishing articles on this subject, there was quite some resistance. People were under the impression that I was abandoning all traditional scientific values. Maybe I did so initially, because I was very enthusiastic about the new discoveries. For thousands of years, herbs have been used to cure certain illnesses without there being a value judgement. Now we can tell exactly why one herb is better than another and why certain herbs are of no influence at all. The components of herbs do tell us something about their medicinal properties but such analysis is never complete, because even if such analysis does seem complete at a certain point, new substances are discovered every day. It is very difficult to determine the medicinal properties of a foodstuff merely by analysing it. Meanwhile, we have succeeded in discovering the link between the energetic and the analytical or material data. According to physics, matter is nothing other than concentrated energy. It is logical that energetic value expresses itself by means of matter. We are familiar with a large number of properties of vitamins, minerals, amino acids, etc. and in fact those properties are determined energetically, since the composition and the shape of a foodstuff are determined genetically. The genetic programme (DNA) is the repository of the biophotons. A simple example can explain this: if a certain foodstuff has a beneficial effect on stomach complaints, that means this foodstuff has a high bio-energetic value on the frequency of the stomach. The medicinal property of a foodstuff is determined genetically and that is why the foodstuff contains the material components that are necessary to realize that property.

Dr Popp rightly claims that the human is a kind of light absorber and that light makes our cells function, but the human is also tied to matter. Energy is converted into matter. That is why the components of a foodstuff still remain of significance. The science of nutrition is not finished because of these new discoveries, but it does gain a new dimension: the energetic aspect.

Everyone understands the word 'intensity'. It is a valuation of energy and force. If a foodstuff indicates a high intensity on the frequency of the liver, that foodstuff has a beneficial effect on the liver. It means the foodstuff can be used to remedy liver complaints. All this is very difficult to imagine, however; that is why we have been studying the exact procedure for this. There is a connection between frequency and wavelength: if we change the wavelength, we also change the frequency – after all, both are invariables. Only amplitude is a variable. We can compare this to the way in which a radio functions. If we change the frequency on the radio, we receive another channel. If we change the frequency on the Lecher antenna, we measure the frequency of another organ. If we turn up the volume on the radio, we increase the amplitude and the sound is amplified. If we measure a high bio-energetic value – that is, a high intensity – it means the amplitude on this frequency is high. If we measure a low value, the amplitude is low. Study Figure 7 for an example.

There are foodstuffs that have a high or a low amplitude on a certain frequency (organ), which means they have a high or a low bio-energetic value (BEV). If a person is healthy, most organs indicate a high bio-energetic value. If the person becomes ill that value drops, either generally or specifically, the latter meaning for a particular organ. A low bio-energetic value on an organ means the amplitude on the frequency of that organ has dropped. If someone wants to increase the amplitude, he or she has to eat something that has a high amplitude on the same frequency. From this we can conclude that the energy that is taken in by the organism is used for energetic recovery. That goes not only for foodstuffs but also for herbs and all other therapies

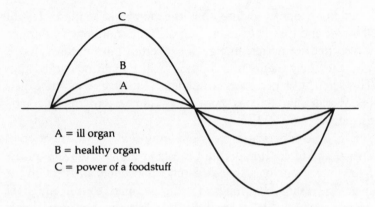

Figure 7 *Diagram of the relationship between bio-energetic value and amplitude*

that are aimed at the body itself, as is known in natural medicine (naturopathy). Inserting an acupuncture needle into an energy point in a meridian is in fact giving an impulse on a certain frequency. Whenever a relaxation therapist uses his or her soft, warm voice to pronounce a relaxation exercise, he or she produces vibrations on a certain frequency, in order to help the subject relax. Pressure point massage and podosegmental re-flexology are in fact used to increase the amplitude on the reflected frequency of the organ concerned. Naturopathy highly values working with energy. Regular medicine, on the other hand, works with means that are not part of the human organism, making use of medication that sets off certain chemical or biochemical reactions to achieve certain effects: pain that disappears, blood vessels that expand, urine that gets another pH value, micro-organisms that are killed, etc. It is an entirely different way not only of curing patients but also of looking at illness and health.

As you can see, the principle of bio-energetics is quite simple: impulses make the amount of energy increase sufficiently for the organism to be able to maintain itself and function optimally.

The actual practice is different, though, because various inhibitions have to be overcome before the energy level can increase.

Cancer, from a Bio-energetic Perspective

There are many cancer theories, which often contradict each other. But cancer is such a complex disease that, in spite of research, no one can give us a clear description of what cancer is. In medical literature (which is quite elaborate nowadays) we can find various descriptions of the properties of certain tumours, cell growth, changes in metabolism, metastasis, mutations, etc. We know a number of mechanisms and the influence of viruses, and we are even familiar with several genetic concepts. What we do not know is what causes cancer. I do not wish to introduce here another cancer theory. All I want to do is to have a look at cancer from the energetic point of view.

Personally, I consider cancer an energetic problem. Human cells function on light energy, and communication plays a large part in that: information is passed and assignments are carried out at the speed of light. That is why a cancer cell starts behaving in another way. The assignment of the cancer cell does not correspond to the assignment of the healthy cells, whose task is to preserve the body. Cancer cells have a destructive influence. The problem is that it is difficult to discover why a cell receives the wrong information. Wrong information may be, for example, the result of defects or substances that cause mutations, like a high dose of radioactivity, chemical substances, asbestos or other dreaded substances that are carcinogenic or aid the development of the cancer. Hereditary material may also be the cause of wrong information – this is called predestination. Cancer is not a hereditary disease, but there are families that are more susceptible than others to cancer.

Cancer may be caused by external influences (exogenous causes), but it may also be caused by internal influences (endogenous causes). But no one knows what exactly causes cancer. In the first chapter I pointed out that cancer is a symptom of degeneration that is caused by an unnatural feeding pattern and an unnatural way of life. If that is correct, we know why humans as a society (mankind) are susceptible to cancer; but then, we still don't know why humans as individuals suffer from it. Meanwhile we *do* know that there are a large number of factors that increase the chance of getting cancer. Research carried out by the American National Cancer Institute in the 1980s shows that farmers who use herbicides (weed killers) on their fields during twenty days or more each year are six times as likely to suffer from lymph node cancer than non-farmers. Farmers who mix the herbicides themselves are eight times as likely to suffer from cancer. Even the length of time that workclothes are worn seemed to have an influence on the origin of cancer. In recent years we have become more and more aware of the fact that environmental pollution, stress, wrong types of food and the many chemical substances that are still used every day have an influence on the origin of cancer. All these negative influences contribute to a drop in levels of bio-energy in humans. When someone is ill, the nature of his or her bio-energy changes. Some possible causes for that are: a shift in waves, a decrease of amplitude (diminution of force), a decrease of electric potential of the cells and depolarization. All these factors interfere with the blood circulation, leading to various obstacles or disturbances. Some researchers assume that all people carry cancer in them, but that it develops in only certain cases. When a person's energy is low, that person is more likely to get cancer, at least if that decrease in energy takes place on the frequency of cancer resistance.

The biological fight against cancer has always paid great attention to metabolism. Dr Moerman even said that a disturbed metabolism was the cause of cancer. Initially, I thought so too, which is why I examined closely foodstuffs with a high bio-energetic value on the frequency of the metabolism. But what I found is that there are many people with metabolic disorders who do not have cancer. Further research allowed me to discover a frequency I later called 'cancer resistance'. I started a systematic search for foodstuffs with a high bio-energetic value on this frequency. Experience has taught me that these foodstuffs indeed have a favourable influence on recovery from cancer. On the other hand I have to admit that metabolism does play an important part, although not a decisive one. A cancer patient cannot recover from cancer simply by improving his or her metabolism.

Every person has a cancer resistance. Cancer resistance must not be confused with general resistance or immunity. The main function of our defence mechanism is to prevent infections. Allergy, for example, is a malfunction of the defence mechanism. Allergy causes the defence mechanism to bolt and react in a chaotic way. The foreign substances that have entered the body are considered dangerous and make the defence mechanism react violently, while in fact there is nothing wrong. Here is an example of an allergy: you are strolling through the woods, enjoying the beauty of nature, and suddenly you have an attack of hay fever, while your companions – who are breathing in the same pollen – do not. With cancer, because a tumour is part of the human body and consists of the same cells even though they behave in a different way, our defence system is not capable of recognizing a tumour as a foreign element. That is why it is so difficult to detect cancer.

Cancer resistance is specific to the disease. If a person's energy on this frequency is high enough, that person does not run the risk of getting cancer. But if his or her energy on this frequency is low, the electric potential of 70–90mV (healthy cell) drops to about 10mV. Nearly every cell has an electric charge. The cellular fluid (cytoplasm) is usually the negative pole and the extracellular fluid is usually the positive pole. In order to maintain an optimal ion composition within the cell, the membrane contains proteins that can transport ions: the ionic pumps. The transportation is not caused by passive diffusion, though; it requires energy from the cell. If the cell cannot produce enough energy, there is depolarization. The depolarization causes the cell to behave in a different way and become a cancer cell. When all is said and done, the only difference between a cancer cell and a healthy cell is its behaviour. Depolarization causes cells to receive the wrong information. Cancer cells have a different polarity and develop according to a programme that does not correspond to the programme that is stored in the DNA. Every living creature is the realization of its own native or natural plan, and from that creature's conception until its death, everything happens according to that plan; but a cancer cell develops according to a different plan, a parallel plan that has nothing to do with our native human plan. Polarity is the direction in which energy moves.

According to chronobiologists, scientists who study the rhythms in living organisms, cancer is caused by disruption of the rhythm of a cell. That more or less summarizes my own opinion. If the electric potential of a cell continues to remain low, the rhythm of that cell is indeed disrupted and that can lead to an overall disruption of the cell. Healthy cells have a constructive function. Cancer cells have a festering and especially a destructive function. Curing cancer means increasing the energy on the frequency of cancer resistance in such a way that the cancer cells are depolarized, so that their energy moves in the right direction again, which also normalizes their rhythm. Within a tumour the depolarization leads to the destruction of cells, which makes the tumour shrivel; that can happen within a very short period of time, which is the strength of the Dries diet. Many cancer patients have started out with a tumour that was not operable. Later their physicians discovered that the tumour had shrivelled. For some patients it took 11 days for that to happen, for others 32 days or 90 days, still others 3 or 4 months. The success of the Dries diet depends on the depolarization. If the depolarization occurs within a short period of time, the oncologist will usually tend to shorten or to suspend the regular treatment, which certainly has great advantages.

There are many factors that may slow down the recovery

process. Cancer is a disease that is different from patient to patient, even if it is the same kind of cancer. Sometimes complications interfere with the recovery process; sometimes the disease develops in such a way that there is no way back. Energetically, this means the amplitude has dropped so drastically that it cannot be increased any more, in spite of strong impulses. The electric potential remains low and there is no depolarization. Personal attitude is of great influence during the recovery process. By fighting the disease with force, a person stimulates his or her own vitality. Vitality is bio-energy. Not only food but also positive thinking can provide us with energy. I will discuss this subject more elaborately later.

There are patients who follow the diet strictly, but who do not manage to benefit from it because of bad digestion or inefficient metabolism. Sometimes the side-effects of the cytostatics have been so destructive that the vitality has been blocked or the organism has been poisoned in such a way that the bio-energy is suppressed by it. In other cases the electro-magnetic pollution in the immediate environment is so serious that the bio-energy cannot be improved. So many obstacles can prevent the energy balance from restoring itself.

The most important aspect of the Dries diet is that it seems to influence the behaviour of the cancer cells, as we have been able to determine with hundreds of cancer patients. Up to now, not a single drug has been able to change the degenerative behaviour of a cancer cell, which is why the tumour always has to be removed by means of surgery, chemotherapy or radiation treatment. The diet allows the body to cure itself. The recovery process is biological and is not brought about by external intervention. This does not mean that regular treatments are not useful. They are, because they take away life-threatening risks.

A small number of foodstuffs have a beneficial bio-energetic value on the frequency of cancer resistance. The Dries diet is based on those foodstuffs, whose bio-energetic value is decisive. The amount of biophotons, determined in the laboratory of Dr Popp, also influences the recovery process but is not the only criterion. An example: a biologically cultivated apple contains many biophotons and is an excellent foodstuff. Nevertheless the biophotons of the apple have a low BEV on the frequency of cancer resistance; in other words, the large amount of biophotons is not enough to increase the cancer resistance. The electric potential cannot be increased by amount, only by intensity. This means that – even if the BEV of a foodstuff on the frequency of cancer resistance is still quite favourable – the amount of biophotons may be very low. This happens, for example, when the foodstuff is unripe, when it has been cultivated using chemical methods, or when it has been poorly stored. In that case the foodstuff is worthless. A high BEV and a sufficient amount of biophotons together, not separately, define the quality of a foodstuff.

Chapter 4

The Composition of the Dries Diet

The keynote of this book was formulated clearly in the previous chapter. If the bio-energy drops, the amplitude on the frequency of cancer resistance also drops, which causes a cell to depolarize and adopt a disparate mode of behaviour. This behaviour leads to the development of a tumour. Because some foodstuffs have a high bio-energetic value on the frequency of cancer resistance, they can be used to restore the energy balance. An important condition, however, is that those foodstuffs should be of good quality. A certain number of nutritional rules have to be taken into account.

If we want to apply the Dries diet correctly, we have to start by dividing the foodstuffs into seven groups, according to their bio-energetic value. The first group consists of the foodstuffs with a very high bio-energetic value. These foodstuffs are essential in order to obtain good results. Groups II and III consist of foodstuffs that are of considerable importance. To sum up, it may be stated that groups I, II and III contain the most important foodstuffs of the diet. The foodstuffs in groups IV, V, VI and VII are considered complementary. Some of these foodstuffs also possess other favourable properties, because they have a high BEV on another frequency – for example, the frequency of the metabolism or the frequency of the defence mechanism. The analytical or material aspect of dealing with foodstuffs must certainly not be neglected; however, in the diet everything is considered holistically, not as separate substances. Some people will say that zinc and selenium are important, but that only makes sense if they are found in foodstuffs with a high bio-energetic value. We use foodstuffs with a high bio-energetic value to provide the necessary nutrients (proteins, fats and carbohydrates), vitamins and minerals; providing light energy also implies providing nutrients.

The foodstuffs from the last groups give the diet variety and make it a lot more attractive – an important aspect we must never lose sight of. A diet always has to be appetizing: if not, the diet's medicinal effect will be hindered.

The next table shows the seven groups into which the foodstuffs are divided. It clearly shows which foodstuffs are part of

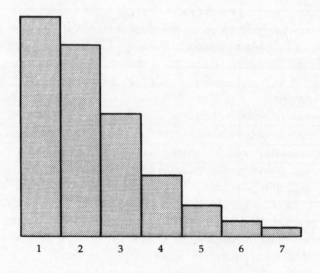

Figure 8 *Chart of the seven groups of the diet*
This chart clearly shows that the diet is based on the first three groups. The diet mainly consists of the foodstuffs that belong to the first three groups. The other foodstuffs have a complementary or supportive function

the diet; only these foodstuffs are to be used. Not only are the foodstuffs divided into seven groups according to their bio-energetic value, but they are also classified under these headings: fruits, nuts/seeds, vegetables and other sources.

Fruits	Nuts/Seeds	Vegetables	Other Sources
Group I			
Pineapple			Pollen
Honeydew melon			Comb honey
Raspberries			
Cactus fruits			
Avocado			
Group II			
Bilberries	Almonds	Chervil	Honey
Kiwi		Mushrooms	
Cherries			
Persimmon			
Apricots			
Yellow Spanish melon			
Melon			
Galea melon			
Mango			
Papaya			
Group III			
Feijoa	Sunflower seeds	All fresh sprouted seeds	Liquid brewer's yeast
Redcurrants	Pumpkin seeds	Germinated wheat	*Panaktiv* – Dr Metz
Blackcurrants			Wheat germ
Strawberries			
Fresh lychees			

Fruits	Nuts/Seeds	Vegetables	Other Sources
Passion fruit			
White grapes			
Red grapes			
Medlar			
Peach			
Group IV			
Ripe banana		Celery	Dextrorotatory yoghurt
Gooseberries		Broccoli	Cottage cheese
Green watermelon		Raw asparagus	Buttermilk
		Watercress	
		Tomato	
		Indian cress	
Group V			
Grapefruit	Sesame seed (black)	White cabbage	Maple syrup
Apple	Hazelnut	Garlic	
Plum	Brazil nut	Green cabbage	
Pear		Onion	
Orange		Shallot	
Mandarins		Shallot shoots	
Lemon		Cauliflower	
Raisins		Chives	
Currants			
Group VI			
	Sesame seed (white)	Cucumber	Egg yolk
		Garden cress	Whey
		Red pepper	*Molkosan*

Fruits	Nuts/Seeds	Vegetables	Other Sources
		Lettuce	
		Gherkin	
		Chicory	
		Lamb's lettuce	
Group VII			
		Herbs (fresh or dried)	Safflower oil
			Corn oil
			Olive oil
			Mayonnaise
			Mustard
			Wine vinegar

Figure 9 Table of the seven groups into which the foodstuffs are divided

The bio-energetic value of a foodstuff is determined genetically, and it is a property of the foodstuff. It is possible that – sooner or later – analytical science will help us discover a number of substances that define this property. In 1990 the American Cancer Research Center examined a number of foodstuffs and discovered substances with a favourable influence on recovery from cancer. In Germany Dr Lothar Schweigerer and Dr Theodore Fotsis of the famous Heidelberg Teaching Hospital carried out similar research; they were mainly interested in fruit and vegetables. In a recent magazine article, nutritionist Prof. Dr Leitzmann of the University of Giessen says the following: 'Phytochemicals or secondary plant substances have been neglected for years; now they are our preferred substances.' But let us not forget that the foodstuffs with favourable effects have been part of the Dries diet for years now: pineapple, broccoli, lemons, garlic, tomatoes, white cabbage and grapes.

In a recent interview that appeared in a local newspaper, Prof.

Dr Jaak Janssens, associated with the cancer research department of the Dr Willems Institute of the University of Diepenbeek (Belgium), claimed that the daily use of 14oz (400g) of fruit reduces the chance of cancer by 50 per cent. He said:

> My conclusions regarding the positive effects of eating fruit and vegetables are based on dozens of scientific reports and studies. These last few years, scientists all over the world have come to the conclusion that fruit and vegetables are the way to prevent several forms of cancer. In seventy per cent of the studies, the conclusion is unanimously positive. In scientific circles, that is an extremely high percentage.

He also emphasized the importance of raw food. According to consumer reports, the consumption of fruit and vegetables in Southern Europe is the same as that in Northern Europe, but in Southern Europe there are remarkably fewer cancer cases. Prof. Dr Janssens noted that that is because people there eat more raw food. He said:

> Research shows that the consumers in Northern Europe mainly eat cooked vegetables. In Southern Europe, food is usually consumed fresh. Apart from that, the international studies mentioned earlier clearly prove that regular consumption of fruit and vegetables discourages the development of cancer.

It has also been known for a long time already that dextrorotary lactic acids have a restraining influence on cancer. Now that more and more scientific research confirms that fruit and vegetables have this restraining influence, confidence in the Dries diet increases from day to day, and it is recommended and applied internationally. Ralph Dochy once did a comparative study on the subject of traditional and energetic herbal medicine, drawing on my research. He concluded that there was a clear parallel. The only difference is that energetic herbal medicine is a lot more accurate and provides us with a better idea of medicinal properties. The same can be said about energetic dietetics.

The Role of Light in the Composition of Foodstuffs

It is interesting to note that, exclusively, the foodstuffs mentioned in the seven groups grow above ground; the seven groups do not include any root crop or tuberous plant. That is not a matter of personal preference though: the selection is based on bio-energetic readings. Bio-energetic value is determined by light. A close look at a plant will reveal an antenna structure; plants are structured in such a way that they are capable of absorbing as much light as possible. Moreover, plants always grow in the direction of the light. We can recognize the antenna structure of the leaves, the branches or twigs and the trunk in almost every plant or tree. Scientists who examine the leaves of trees distinguish 'shadow leaves' and 'sun leaves'. The structure of the sun leaves is completely different from that of the shadow leaves; the shadow leaves are thinner and less mature. Since the discovery of photosynthesis, the influence of light is no longer in doubt.

In a close look at flowers or blossoms, the antenna structure is even more obvious. Flowers and blossoms are tiny biological radars, the structure of whose petals is extremely delicate, almost transparent. The colours are also fascinating, but the delicate structure of the stamens and pistils is incredible. Even more than leaves, flowers are light absorbers and light means energy. Study the inflorescence of a flower, and all will become clear. Flowering season in the vegetable kingdom can be compared to mating season in the animal kingdom. During the flowering season, pollination takes place with the help of insects or the wind. After pollination, the beautiful flowers wither, but the enormous amount of light energy that has been gathered passes to the fruit. In traditional herbal medicine, flowers and blossoms have for years been the most sought-after herbs. Bio-energetic research explains why.

It can be observed that herbs from flowers or blossoms are extremely light compared to herbs from leaves, stalks and roots. Especially roots are very heavy. I have mentioned earlier that matter is in fact concentrated energy, or – in other words – 'condensed' energy. There is a link between energy and matter; the more bio-energy a foodstuff or herb contains, the less matter there is. When energy has materialized, it takes great effort to free that energy from the matter. A herb tea of blossoms needs to brew for only a few minutes for an energy transfer to take place. Herbs from roots are cooked in order to release their medicinal substances, just as we prepare food to be eaten. Fruits, berries, water fruits, nuts, kernels or seeds generally have a very high bio-energetic value on various frequencies. Leaves, stem and stalk plants and bulbous plants usually have a lower bio-energetic value, and the bio-energetic value of root crops is extremely low. Roots grow under the ground and receive light only through the part that grows above the ground. It is logical that we prefer the portions of plants that grow above the ground. That does not mean that carrots, beetroots, turnips and other tuberous plants are bad for our health, but it does take more effort to free the energy that is stored in such plants. Cancer patients need to absorb as much energy as possible, so that their sick bodies use up as little as possible of their energy reserves. Foodstuffs that do not support the recovery process are of no use to them. Root crops are very useful for diabetics, for example, because the sugars – which are stored in the form of starch – are released slowly. But diabetes has another polarity to that of cancer. That is why it is understandable that we need other foodstuffs to cure it. Cancer patients may eat as many root crops or tuberous plants as they want. It will not make them ill, but on the other hand, it will not help them recover either. Some cancer patients are very surprised about that, because beetroot is highly recommended in nearly all books on the biological fight against cancer. Hungarian Dr Firenczi, who examined the beetroot, was thinking in the right direction, though. The group of colouring agents consisting of the anthocyanogens certainly has a favourable influence on cancer. At the university of Graz (Austria), red colouring agents were used in animal experiments and researchers were able to prove their restraining influence on cancer. But betanine – the colouring agents found in beetroot – has a different polarity and is not useful in the fight against cancer. It takes a lot of energy to depolarize betanine. The same colouring agents, but this time with the right polarity, are found in bilberries, red grapes, blackberries and elderberries. Needless to say, *these* colouring agents are suitable. Beetroot does have a number of qualities but does not belong in a cancer diet. Up to now, many researchers have examined the beetroot, which has been used massively in the fight against cancer. Nevertheless, nobody has ever mentioned positive results, not even Dr Firenczi and his fellow countryman E Thyak. The researchers Dr Schmidt, Dr Funk, Dr Trüb, Dr Schulz and others did not obtain positive results either. It is incomprehensible why the use of beetroot is still recommended.

Sometimes they mention that carrots contain significant amounts of beta-carotene or provitamin A, a vitamin to which much attention is given in some cancer diets. Carotene is found in nearly all foodstuffs, but we prefer carotene found specifically in the foodstuffs recommended in this book. We cannot seem to stress it enough: it is never a substance alone that has a medicinal property, it is the substance *in combination with* other substances and compounds in an organic system. From the bio-energetic point of view that is obvious; but for those who think analytically, that is rather a difficult concept to understand.

Genetics

We are on the eve of a genetic revolution. Slowly, a new era in history is dawning. Governments have already invested great amounts of money in research centres. It's now much more likely than ever that we human beings will be able to control nature; genetic engineering seems to make everything possible and to solve all problems. Nevertheless, many people are against genetic engineering, because they fear it will have apocalyptical consequences. Some brilliant successes clear the way for the unknown. The development of nuclear physics entails enormous danger, but even that danger cannot be compared to the danger genetic engineering involves. By changing a gene, certain diseases or hereditary defects can be prevented and that is positive. The people who can be helped by genetic engineering are very grateful for such scientific advances. But they forget what genetic engineering means – that is, changing the life plan of every organism. From the economic point of view, it may be interesting to have a double harvest from one and the same field. But if we decide to do this we have to ask ourselves two questions: 'Is this really necessary?' and 'What will be the quality of genetically engineered foodstuffs?'

When famished primitive man started to chew on the seeds of grasses in his wanderings between the Tigris and the Euphrates, he did not suspect that this was the start of a rapid evolution for mankind. People started grinding the seeds – which we now call grain – in order to obtain flour. With that flour they prepared all kinds of dishes. Suddenly they had found an abundance of food that was easy to store. They discovered that the grains could provide them with a new harvest. That was an early phase in the development of agriculture. But when they harvested the grains, they suffered great losses because the grains were not attached to the ears firmly enough. Biological upgrading made the ears become bigger and contain more grains. The grains stayed in the ears for a longer period of time, so that harvesting them became easier. Those early agriculturalists discovered how to interfere with the genetic plan of the crops in a primitive and quite natural way. Upgrading was a simplified form of genetic engineering. The yields increased, improved, could be stored for a longer period of time and often had a slightly different taste. From the economic and agricultural point of view, it was a true discovery. From the bio-energetic point of view it was a true disaster. We have already pointed out that the history of agriculture is the history of disease. Cancer and other diseases were able to develop in humankind because of human feeding on improved crops.

In the previous chapter it was mentioned that biophotons

are stored in DNA, which also contains hereditary material. Upgrading crops means changing the DNA, which leads to a serious loss of bio-energetic value. If wild bilberries are examined on one hand and cultivated American bilberries on the other, it will be found that the American bilberries are twice the size of the wild bilberries, but that their bio-energetic value is extremely low. Tropical fruits have a high bio-energetic value and that is the reason why tropical fruits are so important in the Dries diet. Until recently, however, tropical fruits were of no economic importance. Tropical fruits grow in the wild. Because they have barely been 'improved', they still possess their unspoilt natural powers. Cactus fruits and bilberries grow in the wild. Pineapples, raspberries and cherries can barely be improved. The fruits that are most commonly used in this diet (first three groups) are quite natural fruits. Apples, oranges, pears and plums have been improved and that is why they belong to the lower-numbered groups. Pollen and comb honey are derived straight from nature. Ever since humans started using agricultural products, they started to suffer from various diseases; to cure those diseases, they started to use herbs medicinally. It must be remembered that medicinal herbs have not been improved – they grow in the wild. The irony of it all: Mankind suffers from diseases because of eating improved foodstuffs and then tries to cure himself by using unspoilt natural plants.

The Dries diet is based on the following reasoning: if we want to give cancer patients a better chance of recovery, if we want to limit the side-effects of heavy therapies, we will have to use the best foodstuffs available. That is why we strongly advise against the use of agricultural products during the recovery process. That may seem weird in the beginning, but once the patient knows our rationale he or she will surely understand. As soon as you have been declared recovered, you are allowed to use small amounts of agricultural products.

The Negative Effects of Agriculture

Mankind lived without knowing cancer for many thousands of years. Like other animals, humans fed themselves on natural plants from unspoilt nature, eating them raw and unprocessed. But when agriculture developed, they started to improve crops and cultivate them in monocultures. That happened in a more or less natural way for centuries. Then scientists discovered which sustaining substances the plants needed and started to imitate those substances in laboratories and to produce them in factories, calling them artificial fertilizers. Artificial fertilizers made agricultural crops row faster, increase in size and produce higher yields. But natural selection disappeared. Normally only unhealthy and weak plants become prey to insects and moulds, or run to weed. That 'problem' was solved by the application of insecticides, fungicides and herbicides. These toxic products inevitably leave residues in foodstuffs.

Many unnatural crops end up in the food industry, nowadays, where they are processed into all kinds of nutritional products. Additives such as colouring agents, preservatives, anti-oxidants, flavourings, emulsifying agents, jelly and thickening agents are in widespread use. Many of these substances have already been taken off the market because of their carcinogenic nature. But how many dangerous substances might there be left? Dangerous substances are only tolerated because there are no substitutes or because substitutes are too expensive.

All these nutritional products are prepared in the kitchen. Not only do we use all kinds of kitchenware to prepare the food, but we also use heat. A lot of food is kept in the freezer for months before we use it. Then we use the microwave-oven to heat it up, or we cook, bake or stew it. We add salt, pepper and nutmeg to give it some taste. In restaurants the food is kept heated for hours and in fast food restaurants it goes straight from the freezer into the microwave.

It seems as if almost no one is concerned with dietary rules. People eat whatever they want, without asking themselves whether their digestive systems can handle it. Most people in Western countries eat about 1,000kg of food a year, not to mention all kinds of sweets, pastries and other snacks that are thought of as treats and not as playing any kind of central role in our daily diet.

Since DNA is the repository for biophotons, it is obvious that every violation of the DNA of a foodstuff has disadvantageous effects on its bio-energetic value. Bio-energetic research has proved that biologically cultivated foodstuffs contain more biophotons than chemically cultivated foodstuffs. Preservation methods for food have also been tested but, unfortunately, each and every method means a loss of bio-energy. Natural and uncontaminated foodstuffs are full of light or photons, whereas industrialized food is synonymous with complete darkness.

No wonder so many scientists claim that – after environmental pollution – industrially processed food is the second most significant cause of cancer. In particular, the influence of the polluted environment on food should not be neglected. Just think of the heavy metals with which industry pollutes the soil: cadmium, arsenic, lead, etc. Apart from that there is also air pollution caused by exhaust fumes of cars, central heating, industry, etc.

We humans are sufficiently aware of all these dangers, but we have become indifferent and/or powerless towards them. 'What can I do?' everyone says, even though that's not an excuse. But when someone is struck by cancer, the need for clean food suddenly increases. The Dries diet tries to offer you food that is part of uncontaminated nature.

Meat

It's quite evident that cancer patients acquire an aversion to meat soon after the development of their illness. That is why very few cancer diets allow meat. Man is not a meat-eater *by nature* – that notion is generally accepted by science. Man has *learned* to eat meat, just as he has learned to eat fish, bread and pulses. Nutritionists often say that man has expanded his food range during the course of history, but they forget to mention that he has done so at a disadvantage to his own health. Meat has not been a subject of discussion for quite a while now. The widespread consumption of meat in the West, which started around 1950, has been dealt a heavy blow recently. The discussions regarding the use of hormones and especially of mad cow disease (BSE) have changed the eating pattern of the Westerner. However, one thing only is sure: we do not really need meat. After all, we are not natural meat-eaters. Meat is a rather unhygienic foodstuff that spoils easily, and that is nearly always infected by bacteria, even though there are laws that limit the admissible amount of bacteria.

Because man is not by nature a meat-eater, his digestive system is not suitable for processing meat. Meat is very difficult to digest: it takes a lot of energy to free the substances of which meat consists. Bowel movement becomes difficult and there is putridity in the bowels resulting in malodorous flatulence. There are many meat-eaters among cancer patients. Polluted intestines not only mean an overburdened liver, but also polluted bodily fluids: intra- and extracellular fluids are poisoned, and that has a direct influence on the life of cells. Meat is an important supplier of proteins, but the human animal needs very few proteins – at least, if the correct proteins are used.

Raw and Unspoilt Foodstuffs

Danish Dr Nolfi (1881–1957) suffered from breast cancer herself. She managed to overcome her illness by eating nothing but raw foods. 'We have to eat our food as nature provides it,'[1] was her point of view. She was strongly influenced by the ideas of Dr Bircher Benner, a famous Swiss nutritionist. This famous

[1] Quoted in Jan Dries, *Kanker genezen volgens de Dr. Nolfi-therapie*, Nieuw Leven, Arinus, Genk, 1990, p. 65.

naturopath said: 'Food is sublimed solar energy.'[2] He based this statement on research similar to that of Dr Gurwitsch. Now we know with absolute certainty that foodstuffs are highly significant suppliers of light. Dr Nolfi's work is of great importance because she experimented with raw food diets for years. She did that at her health resort called 'Humlegaarde', near Copenhagen. Furthermore, her own illness and that of many fellow-sufferers made her realize the absolute necessity of raw food during the treatment of cancer. She says: 'The best food is the living food that has not undergone any treatment, regardless of what nature.'[3] Food has to be eaten uncooked, if at all possible. Cooking food means destroying its vitality and that has a disastrous effect on the important substances the food contains, such as vitamins, enzymes and minerals. The use of living food allows us to increase our strength and our stamina when we perform heavy physical labour. Moreover, the use of living food (more than with any other food) increases our sense of initiative and vitality when we perform spiritual labour.

What Dr Nolfi wrote with so much conviction can now be proved by bio-energetic research. My own experience, with hundreds of cancer patients who started using raw food, confirms the high value of raw food. If a cancer patient decides to apply the Dries diet, his or her blood analysis will show remarkable improvement within a relatively short period of time. The vitality of the patient will increase in spite of the heavy treatments. One cancer patient told me she noticed that she was skiing a lot better during her last winter holiday than she was during the years before she became ill. The advantages of raw food should not be doubted. Dietetics tells us the seriousness of a loss of nutrients resulting from a high preparation temperature. People are very concerned about vitamins and minerals nowadays, but still they do not realize that – by heating food – vitamins and minerals are destroyed or made inactive. From the

[2] Quoted in Jan Dries, *Voedingstherapie*, Arinus, Genk, 1990, p. 40.
[3] Quoted in Jan Dries, *Kanker genezen volgens de Dr. Nolfi-therapie*, Nieuw Leven, Arinus, Genk, 1990, p. 88.

bio-energetic point of view, heat only brings chaos. Moreover, heat makes the BEV drop to such a level that it cannot even be measured any more. We cannot say that cooked food is worthless, but it is certainly inferior: the body has to use a lot of energy to get the useful substances out of it. That is why people need more and more food to provide them with the most basic nutrients. We have been neglecting the importance of enzymes in food for much too long; enzymes are bio-catalysts that are very important during digestion. The body itself produces a large number of digestive enzymes, but normally foodstuffs also contain enzymes. Unfortunately, heat destroys those enzymes.

People who follow the Dries diet eat exclusively raw food for the first three months, or sometimes for a little bit longer. This is the only way for them to absorb unspoilt proteins, sugars, fats, vitamins, minerals, enzymes and other substances, all of which provide them with large amounts of biophotons with a high intensity. And that is exactly the strength of the Dries diet. The Dries diet is so simple and its composition so natural that the dieter spontaneously applies the rules of correct food combining. It provides a perfect acid-base balance, which makes it impossible to break the rules of correct food combining. When one patient told his oncologist that he was following the Dries diet, the latter said: 'If everyone followed such a diet, we would certainly have a lot fewer problems.'

Chapter 5

The Dries Diet Food Groups

The Dries diet consists of a limited number of foodstuffs. That restriction is the result of a strict selection. Only foodstuffs with a high bio-energetic value on the frequency of cancer resistance are qualified. These foodstuffs are mainly found in the first three groups. The last four groups consist of foodstuffs that do have a favourable influence on the recovery process, but not to the same extent as the foodstuffs in the first three groups. The seventh group consists of a number of foodstuffs that are meant to make the diet more attractive. They do not have a direct influence on the recovery process, but they are not harmful either.

The chart that presents an overall picture of the foodstuffs (see Figure 9, pp. 55–7) clearly shows that fruits – that is, mainly tropical fruits – are the most important foodstuffs. Basically, the Dries diet is a fruit diet that is supplemented with vegetables, nuts, seeds and a few other sources. The most important foodstuffs of each group are described here, with those having the highest bio-energetic value given first. Their nutritional value will be discussed later.

Group I

The pineapple

The pineapple is the most essential foodstuff in the Dries diet. It is at the top of the list and on the menu every day during the first period. A fascinating fruit that is popular all over the world, it belongs to the Bromeliaceae, a family of plants with thousands of members, but is the only one of those to produce an edible fruit. The pineapple has its origins in South America; the name means 'precious fruit'. The English call it pineapple because it looks like a pine cone. The pineapple plant usually reaches a height of about 32in (80cm). It consists of a rosette of long, narrow leaves. When the plant is 15 to 20 months old, a ligneous stalk grows from its centre. On that stalk, hundreds or more flowers develop. Each flower develops into a small fruit. The various fruits grow towards one another, until they form a conical false fruit; the separate fruits can be recognized by the shoots on the outside of the pineapple. A pineapple plant in bloom can be compared to a radar station with 100 or more radar units. It attracts a lot of light; thus the pineapple has an extremely high bio-energetic value. Unlike most fruits, the pineapple has a very difficult time ripening after it has been cut off the stalk, at which time the ripening process stops. That is why we prefer pineapples that have been transported by aeroplane, which we call 'aeroplane pineapples' or 'sun-ripened pineapples' as opposed to 'boat pineapples', which are picked unripe so that they can withstand long sea journeys. In order to encourage the ripening process of these pineapples, they are usually kept in plastic bags together with ripe bananas. Needless to say, these pineapples will never have the quality of sun-ripened pineapples. There are various kinds of pineapple and almost all can be used, the exception being mini-pineapples: these are planted too close to each other, and so cannot find enough food and are not able to mature. Pineapple is available throughout the entire year because it is imported from different producing areas each time. The high season of the pineapple is from September to December. It is not, however, always easy to find a suitable quality.

The cactus fruit

The family of the Cactaceae consists of about 2,000 varieties. The fruits of a number of cacti, also called *cotyledons*, are edible. The cactus fruit that is part of our diet is the prickly pear or *opuntia*. The prickly pear grows in the wild and can reach a maximum height of about 10ft (3m). In spring, it grows yellow flowers. In summer and autumn, those flowers develop into large cotyledons which initially are green; but during their ripening process, their colour changes from yellow to orange and bright red and finally to reddish brown. Just like the plant itself, the fruit also has spines. It is a watery fruit with a refreshing taste, and its small seeds are also edible. The high bio-energetic value is a consequence of the unspoilt nature of the cacti.

The avocado

The avocado belongs to the laurel family, the Lauraceae, and there are many sorts and varieties. The avocado tree has its origins in Central and South America: the original Aztec name for the avocado fruit was 'Ahuacatl', which can be translated as 'butter from the woods'. Unlike the other fruits in the diet, the avocado is a high-fat fruit (23 per cent). It contains less water (68 per cent) than other fruits. The avocado plays an important part in the diet because it supplies fats, proteins and of course calories. To make the flesh of the fruit more digestible, you can add lemon juice to it. All varieties are suitable, as long as they are very ripe.

The raspberry

The raspberry belongs to the family of the rosaceous plants (the Rosaceae), a family to which 28 well-known and less known fruits belong. The raspberry is a very soft fruit that may be yellow, red, pink, orange, brown or black, dependent on the variety. Raspberries are very perishable fruits, and are available from June to September.

The honeydew melon

This melon is a member of the cucumber family (the Cucurbitaceae). It is the fruit of a climbing or creeping herbaceous plant. The fruit has a relatively high sugar content, which explains its sweet taste and its name. The honeydew melon has a rather high bio-energetic value, and thus belongs to the first group. There are different varieties, but the Cavallions are the most popular.

Pollen

Bees collect microscopic pollen grains from flowers and blossoms and turn them into little balls, which they transport between their legs. The quality of the pollen depends on its origin -- that is, which flower it came from -- and the climatological circumstances. Pollen consists of a large number of substances and has a wide range of medicinal properties. Nevertheless some precautions have to be taken. People who suffer from hayfever must not use pollen because of possible allergic reactions. When pollen is to be used, it is also advisable to check blood pressure, which in some people increases when they use pollen.

Comb honey

Bees possess nectaries that produce honey, which is collected in combs. The bee-keeper takes the honey out of the combs and keeps it in pots. The advantage of comb honey is that it's unspoilt – the combs are sealed in such a way that oxidation is ruled out. Comb honey is available in most natural food shops and honey shops; very often it comes from New Zealand. The quality of the comb honey is determined by means of its origin. Comb honey is very sweet and has a very high bio-energetic value.

Group II

This group consists of a large number of foodstuffs of which the bio-energetic value is slightly less high than that of the foodstuffs in group I. Nevertheless the foodstuffs of group II remain very important.

The bilberry

The bilberry belongs to the heather family (the Ericaceae) and is indigenous. The red colouring agent of this wild fruit has a restraining influence on cancer. The bilberry also has a favourable influence on the intestines and is used in case of diarrhoea when all else fails.

The kiwi

The kiwi is a fruit that belongs to the family of the climbers (the Actinidiae). It is mainly found in East Asia and in the Himalayas, and has its origins in South China. As a consumer good, the kiwi owes its existence to the growers of New Zealand who started exporting the kiwi after World War II. A kiwi is ripe when its flesh yields to soft pressure. The kiwi is full of vitamin C and also contains a protein-separating enzyme.

The cherry

The cherry is an occidental fruit with a very high bio-energetic value, probably because the cherry is so hard to improve. The cherry possesses various medicinal properties. All varieties are useful, as long as they are very ripe.

The persimmon

The persimmon is a fruit that has the shape and colour of a tomato. The stalk ends in a four-labiate calyx. It belongs to the family of the Ebenaceae and has its origins in China and Japan, and is now cultivated in the Mediterranean region. The persimmon has a very high tannic acid (tannin) content, but that disappears as soon as the fruit is completely ripe. While the fruit remains unripe it has a bitter, sour taste that makes tongue and palate contract in an unpleasant way. But when the fruit is ripe, it has a sweet, aromatic flavour. Persimmons have to be eaten ripe. That is why it is advisable to let them ripen in the presence of other fruits. (The sharon fruit is a persimmon that has lost not only its core and seeds because of biological upgrading, but also its tannic acid. It has a very low bio-energetic value and is not part of this diet.)

The apricot

The Hunzas – a tribe that lives in the Himalayas and that does not know any illnesses – consider the apricot so important that a widow always inherits an apricot tree. The apricot tree has beautiful white blossoms and produces tasty fruits. The apricot belongs to the family of rosaceous plants. The apricot has to be eaten ripe in order for it to be juicy.

The melon

Because the Dries diet pays a lot of attention to water balance, it includes a lot of water fruits. The honeydew melon belongs to group I. Other melons, such as the yellow Spanish melon, the Galea melon and the ordinary or Dutch melon, belong to group II. The popular green watermelon belongs to group IV.

The mango

The mango belongs to the family of the smoketrees (the Anacardiaceae). In the tropics, the mango is the second most popular tropical fruit, after the banana. There are several varieties. The colour of a ripe mango varies either from green to yellow or from orange to crimson. The flesh of the mango is orange-yellow and has a very soft structure. A mango of good quality contains hardly any fibres. The mango has a large stone and a turpentine-like aroma. Mangos also ripen easily after being picked.

The papaya

Sometimes the papaya is also called tree-melon because its composition corresponds to that of a melon. Papayas have a very low calorific value. They contain little sugar and much water. They grow on almost leafless trees, always forming small groups. There are several varieties with different shapes and sizes. The papaya is famous for its protein-separating enzyme *papain*. We prefer the use of sun-ripened fruits.

Almonds

An almond is a very special nut with very positive qualities; it is the sweet almond to which we refer. Almonds have a rich composition and also possess medicinal properties. They have a favourable influence on the calcium balance and on the defence mechanism. In this diet they are specifically used to level the mineral balance.

Chervil

Chervil is a vegetable with a remarkably delicate structure and a wonderful aroma. Of all vegetables, chervil has the highest bio-energetic value. That is why chervil belongs to group II. Chervil is in fact an aromatic herb.

Mushrooms

Mushrooms are fungi with a very light structure. The function of fungi in nature is to convert organic material into inorganic material. In other words their job is to get rid of rubbish. During this clear-out, the biophotons that remain in the waste products are recycled, which is why fungi still manage to have a rather favourable bio-energetic value. That high bio-energetic value is mainly found in the cap of the mushroom, but that doesn't mean you have to throw away the stalk. Raw mushroom is a natural antibiotic.

Honey

Because the most common honey varieties have a lower bio-energetic value than comb honey, they belong to group II. When honey is being purchased, special attention has to be paid to its quality. Pure, natural honey has a large number of favourable qualities. The presence of hibin guarantees strong antiseptic effects. Honey is a natural antibiotic, and its high sugar content has a calming effect.

Group III

The Feijoa

The Feijoa is a less known tropical fruit. It belongs to the large myrtle family (the Myrtaceae), the same family to which the guava belongs. It is a round, elongated fruit with a length of 1⅕–4in (3–10cm) and a diameter of ¾–2in (2–5cm). The skin is green and the flesh cream-coloured. Its taste can be compared to that of a pineapple.

The red- and the blackcurrant

Both currants are part of the diet. They belong to the *Savifrage* family, the same family to which the gooseberry belongs. The blackcurrant has a very typical aroma that not everyone appreciates. Currants contain good amounts of vitamin C. The red colouring agent of redcurrants is said to have a restraining influence on cancer. Redcurrants are very tasty and have many positive qualities.

The strawberry

The strawberry is a false fruit and belongs to the family of the rosaceous plants, just as the raspberry. The strawberry lacks sugar and that is why it has a low calorific value. The strawberry also has many positive qualities.

The lychee

The lychee is a very desirable fruit in China and in other tropical countries. Lychees belong to the family of the Sapindaceae. In recent years, they have been available fresh. They have a thin, red shell that is easy to remove. The flesh surrounds a large, brown stone and is juicy and tasty. In the Aki, you will find a pink, poisonous membrane between the flesh and the stone. The Aki is not sold in this part of the world.

The passion fruit

This is the fruit of the passion flower. There are three varieties but the purple variety or the yellow variety is the most popular one. A ripe passion fruit can be recognized by its shrivelled skin. The flesh consists of a greenish, juicy pulp that contains edible seeds. The fruit is usually cut in half and then spooned out. The passion fruit has a very delicate aroma.

The white and the red grape

The grape is one of the oldest cultivated plants and belongs to the vine family (Vitaceae). Research has shown that grapes contain ellagin acid, one of the very highly recommended phyto-chemicals with a restraining influence on cancer.

The medlar

The medlar is an occidental fruit and belongs to the family of rosaceous plants. Its skin is quite hard and feels rough. The fruit contains five gritty stones. Medlars have to be very ripe before you eat them. Some people claim they have to be rotten first, but that is not true. After they've been picked, however, they must be further ripened.

The peach

The peach can be compared to the apricot. If it is to be eaten juicy, it must be eaten when very ripe. However, the nectarine – a mutant of the peach – is not part of the diet because it has a much lower bio-energetic value.

Sunflower seeds

A sunflower always grows facing the sun, and that is why it contains good amounts of solar energy. That solar energy is stored in the seeds, which are quite soft and can be easily chewed. They also have a high nutritional value.

Pumpkin seeds

Pumpkin seeds are often used to remedy prostate complaints. Just like sunflower seeds they are very nutritious. They are also important in the fight against prostate cancer.

Wheat germ

This is the germ of wheat collected during grinding. Because wheat germ becomes rancid quite easily, it is fermented or stabilized as soon as possible. One needs 220lb (100kg) of wheat to produce 9oz (250g) of wheat germ. That is why wheat germ is very concentrated and full of vitamins, minerals and nutrients. Wheat germ is a natural supplement.

Germinated wheat

Wheat grains can be germinated in bowls and plates that are especially designed for that purpose. Every wheat grain produces a germ which is, however, less concentrated than the wheat grain. If you are familiar with germinating wheat, you can use germinated wheat.

Sprouts

You can let all kinds of seeds germinate. Sprouts are very young plants and therefore belong to the group of vegetables. They have a very high bio-energetic value and can be used in the diet daily. Only the sprouts of pulses and soybean sprouts are not recommended and are not part of this diet.

Liquid brewer's yeast

Liquid brewer's yeast is a waste product from breweries. It is full of vitamin B but also contains valuable proteins and of course yeasts. It has to be seen as a natural supplement or support of the diet. Liquid brewer's yeast is used in small amounts, usually separated from meals (one or two 150cc glasses a day). Brewer's yeast cannot be used during the summer because it ferments very quickly. Only brewer's yeast prepared according to traditional fermentation methods is suitable; brewer's yeast tablets are considered to have no value.

Panaktiv – Dr Metz

This is a liquid yeast with more or less the same properties as liquid brewer's yeast. For some people this yeast is easier to obtain, especially when there is no old-fashioned brewery in the neighbourhood.

Group IV

The banana

I'm sure everyone knows the banana. The ripe banana has the highest sugar content of all fruits and therefore is the most nutritious fruit. The banana possesses an excellent potassium-sodium balance (proportion) and that is very important in a cancer diet. It contains serotonin, a neurotransmitter that makes nerve contact possible. (Lack of serotonin in the brain can result in depression and suicidal tendencies.) Because of rigorous biological upgrading, the banana has lost its high bio-energetic value, but it remains an important fruit. You can let bananas ripen by keeping them in a plastic bag together with apples. Bananas are ripe when they start to show tiny brown spots. Many people experience a feeling of hunger when they switch over to the Dries diet, which means that their digestive system and their metabolism have not yet adjusted to the diet. For them, a ripe banana is the best solution, especially if they eat it very slowly.

Gooseberries

Gooseberries have to be eaten ripe. They contain important fruit acids and have a favourable influence on the intestines.

The green melon

The green melon is an important water supplier, and filters the groundwater through its roots and stalks. The water of the green melon has an energetic charge and is an excellent thirst-quencher. Like other melons, the green melon is not very nutritious.

The brazil nut

Like all nuts, the brazil nut is very nutritious. It contains several minerals, fats and high-quality proteins. The brazil nut also contains selenium, a mineral that is important in the fight against cancer.

The coconut

Of all foodstuffs, the coconut contains the largest amount of selenium. Selenium is an important component of the enzyme glutathionperoxydase, which is found in most human tissues. This enzyme plays an important part in the metabolic process of polyunsaturated fatty acids and prevents the development of free radicals: that is why the coconut is essential to this diet.

Vegetables

It has probably been noted by now that chervil is the only vegetable in the first three groups. The composition of a mushroom is very similar to that of a vegetable, but still it belongs to the group of yeasts. Bio-energetic research shows us that vegetables have a much lower value than fruits and nuts, which is logical since fruits (fruits, berries, nuts, seeds, pips) always grow from flowers and blossoms. Moreover, humans are considered fruit-eaters or *frugivores* and fruits should constitute their basic food.

Vegetables take only second place in the Dries diet. Because vegetables are easy to grow and inexpensive, and because there are so many varieties, we feel we can also recommend their use. Because humans are not vegetable-eaters or *herbivores*, a lot of people have difficulties digesting raw vegetables. And as we all know, undigested leftovers cause fermentation and other digestive problems. The reason why I allow vegetables to be part of my diet is that a lot of cancer patients, especially during the first stage of the diet, prefer the powerful aroma of vegetables to the sweet taste of fruit. Moreover, the vegetables I have selected all have a number of other qualities too. Tomatoes (really, in any case, a fruit not a vegetable), broccoli, white cabbage and garlic contain phytochemicals or cancer-restraining substances. Watercress, celery, asparagus, tomatoes and broccoli have been placed in the fourth group because of their bio-energetic value.

Vegetables are absolutely not an essential part of this diet. If it is difficult for you to digest them, you can leave them out completely or limit yourself to small amounts.

Dairy products

Older diets pay a lot of attention to milk and dairy products. The Nolfi diet, for example, recommends 2⅝–3½pt (1.5–2 litres) of milk a day. But because a lot of people are allergic to milk and dairy products, the use of these products in the domain of health treatments has dropped significantly. People often ask me why I have kept three dairy products in my diet. My explanation is quite simple: bio-energetic research indicates that these three dairy products (cottage cheese, yoghurt and buttermilk) are suitable to belong to group IV. They are not important for the diet but they are of practical use. Patients appreciate it if they are allowed to mix fruit with yoghurt and they enjoy drinking buttermilk. The fermented dairy products we mention here are easy to digest. The most important protein in milk is called *casein*, the structure of which is unique and loose and can be compared to the structure of snowflakes. Moreover, casein contains ten times the amount of water found in other proteins. The favourable influence of lactic acids in the fight against cancer has been proved over and over again. Dextrorotary yoghurt is an ideal foodstuff to support the intestinal flora. Once again, I would like to add that dairy products are absolutely not essential. If the dieter does not like milk or does not wish to drink milk for ethical reasons, milk can be left out of the diet.

Group V

Group V consists of a number of fruits such as oranges, mandarins, apples, pears, plums and grapefruit. The orange has a number of good qualities but, just like the other fruits in this group, it has a low bio-energetic value because it has been upgraded. All these fruits are allowed, but their medicinal value is limited. They should be considered as supplements.

Black sesame seed (not roasted) and hazelnuts also belong to this group. Other members of this group are: garlic, onions and shallots, mainly because of their antiseptic effects, white cabbage, green cabbage and cauliflower because they contain phytochemicals. Maple syrup, raisins and currants can be used as sweeteners.

Group VI

This group consists of a number of popular vegetables that can be used as supplements. Egg yolk is often recommended because it contains the vitamin choline and because it stimulates the defence mechanism. Since this diet is nearly cholesterol-free, the small amount of cholesterol in the form of one or two egg yolks will not do any harm; indeed, cholesterol also has good qualities, especially where the sex glands are concerned. Whey, *Molkosan* and sauerkraut can also be used in small amounts because they contain lactic acid.

Group VII

This group consists of a number of foodstuffs that are not really necessary, but nevertheless indispensable for preparing a meal. Avocados, nuts and seeds are the best suppliers of fat, because they contain fat in an organic structure. But if a sauce or a mayonnaise is to be prepared, cold vegetable oil, wine vinegar or lemon juice can be used. If the dieter wants to add some whipped cream to the fruit (especially when only just starting to apply the diet), there is no objection to that. The presence of whipped cream slows down the digestion and therefore also improves it. The same goes for vegetables. Some people refuse to use mayonnaise or vinaigrette because they want to keep what they eat natural, but that is not very wise. These sauces are not only meant to make the meal more tasty, but also to improve digestion.

Chapter 6

Beginning the Diet

Cancer patients who are confronted with the Dries diet for the first time are always startled. 'Is that possible? Is that really possible with such a diet?' are their first reactions. Immediately a lot of questions arise. We admit it is an unfamiliar diet, especially for anyone not conversant with natural foodstuffs, but it does have an attractive aspect. Many people apply this diet not only because they hope it will give them a better chance of recovery, but also because it allows them to participate in the recovery process in an active way.

The diet enables cancer patients to do something themselves. During a recent conference in Antwerp that was largely dedicated to the Dries diet, and during which several ex-cancer patients came to testify about their recovery, it suddenly dawned on me that ex-cancer patients value their active participation in the recovery process very highly. One of the ex-cancer patients said: 'If a physician now tells me my condition has improved, I know I have myself, my own dedication, to thank for that.' Many cancer patients rebel against this polluted world, the commercialized food and the artificial way of life, both consciously and unconsciously. They are searching for another value in life. Life-threatening diseases such as cancer, AIDS and ALS always involve a lot of emotion. They make people think about existential questions, about life and death, about the meaning of life and about suffering. The moment the doctor mentions the diagnosis 'cancer', the patient's world is crushed and he or she is overwhelmed with uncertainty, losing all perspective about the future as if that world were going to end tomorrow.

When I found out that an acquaintance of mine had cancer, I went to visit him. This man, whose prognosis was very bad, was sitting in his chair, staring aimlessly. He barely had the courage to engage in conversation. Because of his condition, the doctors had shattered his last hope. They had told him that he had only three months left to live, at the most. He was only 55 years old. I did not want to raise false hopes. I did not want to make idle promises I wouldn't be able to keep anyway. But on the other hand, I could not just leave someone in such a desperate situation. Even though we needed an interpreter to communicate, we had an in-depth, encouraging discussion. There was a light at the end of the long, dark tunnel and that light grew bigger every day. The diet was his only hope; but he managed to hang on to that hope. He was extremely brave in his suffering, and was still able to spend many wonderful days with his loving family and – against all odds – survived for 15 months instead of 3, precisely a year longer than expected. The diet had not only prolonged his life; it had also made it more bearable and pleasant. He had started to look at his illness from a different point of view and had spent the rest of his life in a very conscious and intense way.

Luckily, not everyone finds himself in that man's situation. But everyone who is confronted with cancer knows the feeling of having to live without a future. It is an unbearable, depressing feeling. A patient is powerless in dealings with the medical world, from which he or she expects too much anyway; is not prepared; does not know what is going to happen, how to go on, who can give support and counsel; wants to do something on his or her own but does not know what. That is why a first conversation about the Dries diet is so important. The moment a patient makes an appointment with me to talk about the diet, there is already a certain willingness. It means he or she is ready to consider new possibilities. The diet gives cancer patients the opportunity to contribute to their own recovery process, to take an active part in it.

I have often met caner patients who were like defenceless wrecks, discouraged and disappointed. They bottled everything up: sorrow, fear and despair. And yet I found a little bit of gameness in every one of those people; the survival instinct prevails, in spite of everything. Very often relatives encourage cancer patients to take action. One should never lose heart: 'While there is life, there is hope,' the old saying goes.

I always notice that cancer patients are very brave, that it is easy for them to discuss their illness, sometimes even easier than for their relatives to do so. They are always in search of certainty, security, guarantees, which – unfortunately – nobody can give them. I can only rely on my experience with hundreds of cancer patients. If someone follows my diet for three months, any oncologist will be able to determine an improvement or at least a stabilization in that person. For some people that improvement is surprising; for others it may be a stabilization of the condition; and for still others a deterioration of the condition. The Dries diet has a positive influence on recovery from cancer and it supports regular treatment very well. The Dries diet does not have any disadvantages. There is no risk of malnutrition because the diet contains all the essential and non-essential nutrients the human needs. We can easily meet the standards of traditional dietetics with this diet, even though we do have alternative opinions on several subjects. The Dries diet only has advantages. It is a pity that some people refuse to follow this diet, considering all the advantages it entails. The Dries diet cleanses the whole organism; it improves digestion and the metabolism; it takes care of water regulation; it strengthens defence mechanisms and fights cancer. These curious effects are due to the high bio-energetic value of the selected foodstuffs.

Not everyone finds it easy to take the first step towards the Dries diet. Many similar diets have fallen short of expectations, in spite of promising reports. Most of those diets are now quite dated, having been developed during a time when we didn't yet know much about cancer and nutrition. They do bring about an improvement in the general condition of the patient, but they barely influence the cancer.

A number of alternative physician encouraged me to develop a diet more powerful than the existing diets. With the help of bio-energetic research, that was possible. I can understand why people are quite sceptical about cancer diets. Apart from the Dries diet, not a single diet produces large-scale improvements. That is why the other diets can only cure a limited number of patients. And even then we are talking about isolated cases. For ten years we have experimented, counselled hundreds of cancer patients, studied the evolution of their illness, constantly adapted and improved the diet. Now that we have proof of the positive results, now that we have evidence that the diet works for more or less everyone, we are trying to give it the publicity it deserves. The Dries diet gives hope to thousands of cancer patients.

Unfortunately, many people still doubt the possibilities of nutritional therapy, even though there is a close link between food and health. Besides, it takes a lot of effort to switch to another diet. Food has to do with taste, tradition and habit and it is not that easy to abandon existing concepts. People tend to experience initial resistance, and that has to be overcome. A cancer patient told me this:

> I have to go to the hospital regularly. Whenever I'm in the waiting room of the oncology department I feel as if I'm surrounded by people who've escaped from a concentration camp. They look pale and faceless, skinny and especially very indifferent. Ever since I started following the Dries diet, I feel like I'm flourishing. My face has a healthy colour again and my muscles have strength again. I've turned into a completely different person. A lot of my fellow sufferers ask me what has made me change in such a short period of time and I'm always proud to tell them about the diet I'm following. Many of them have asked me for your address.

Unfortunately, none of those people came to consult me. They witnessed the improvement with their own eyes, they envied the positive development, and still they did not follow the example. I understand the point of view of these and many others, and I know their objection. They all think: 'That is not possible. There is no way food can have such positive results.' But it is possible. I see it happen every day. And even more important is the fact that oncologists also notice the improvement in our patients. It has been years since a certain patient told her physician she was following a diet. He admitted that her condition was improving a lot better than the condition of his other patients. He reassured her: 'Just continue following your diet.' At a certain point that same physician suspected two other patients were also following the diet. He was right. Their exceptional improvement had betrayed them. Patients who follow the Dries diet experience a completely different recovery process. They recover more rapidly and they feel more vigorous. Their blood analysis shows different results and they are less likely to relapse. One day a medical specialist of a famous teaching hospital invited me for a visit. He told me the following: 'I invited you because I felt I needed to speak with you urgently. We can tell exactly which patients follow your diet. They catch the eye because they are so vital, because they recover so quickly after chemotherapy and especially because their recovery process is very different from that of other patients.' He was completely convinced of the importance of the Dries diet. 'But', he added, 'the oncologists are not open to it yet.' He himself was a haematologist.

Sometimes patients ask their physician whether he or she objects to them following a diet, since there once were many physicians who mocked diets. Luckily that is not the case any more. I still remember the case of Antje Mahler, a patient who had a tumour under the collarbone. When she started following the diet, she was full of enthusiasm. But when she told her physician about it, he immediately answered: 'No one has ever been cured by a diet before.' Eleven days later, that same physician was unable to locate the tumour. He asked Antje which diet she was following. She smiled and said: 'No one has ever been cured by a diet before.' The physician apologized and mentioned he was going to retire within a couple of months. 'But I want to see you as my last patient,' he said. 'You are the touchstone of my career.' In his whole career as an oncologist, he had never seen anything like this.

Some physicians think of a diet as a kind of psychotherapy or an alternative for Lourdes or Fatima. Suggestion or the power of thought should not be underestimated. Some people recover by following a diet that has no nutritional value at all. In such cases, the diet is the means that makes the suggestion possible. In China they sometimes feed rice with fried worms to ill people. Of course the Chinese also have an aversion to that. But whoever is convinced that he or she will recover by eating such a dish, will indeed recover. Suggestion can never be eliminated and it is not necessary to eliminate it. Nevertheless the Dries diet is not based on suggestion. It is based on nutritional research. Luckily, more and more physicians are convinced the Dries diet really works. They see the remarkable improvements in patients who have discontinued all medical treatments and who follow nutritional therapy only. Some of those patients had to discontinue other treatments because they cold not bear them any more or because the chemotherapy did not produce any results. Even those patients stay alive, their condition improves and many of them recover in spite of the fact that they have discontinued all medical treatments. I cannot understand why on earth people should continue to doubt the diet any longer. Patients often tell me that their physician reacts in a positive way, not only to the diet but also to the results. When I ask them why they are not spreading the good news, they always tell me they do not have time, they are too busy at the hospital, etc. There is a lot of contradiction in medical circles. In one book people are warned against using a diet and even mention possible dangers, and in another book they are told that industrialized food is responsible for the increase in cancer cases. One physician wants them to stick to traditional food, while another tells them to find another way to prevent cancer. A professor from a famous university advised me to have my diet launched by physicians. 'It will create more confidence,' he said. I disagree with that. Cancer patients have to opt for this diet out of free will and conviction. With their remarkable improvements, they have to convince the physicians the diet works, and not the other way round. I recommend my diet to each and every cancer patient. The Dries diet will help them. It will not only free them of their disease but it will also turn them into different people. People often say: 'A cancer patient will never be the same again.' I cannot agree with that either. Many cancer patients have told me: 'Life has become very different, more conscious, more intense.' Cancer patients experience life, illness and health in a completely different way. They discover new values in life and are able to enjoy the simple things in life.

Be honest, though: people choose to follow this diet because they do not want to die. But only few, however, are aware of the fact that the diet can have a strong influence on life in general. All the more reason why people should choose to follow this diet. Unfortunately, not everyone feels that way. I was once consulted by a man who suffered from larynx cancer. He said the diet did not appeal to him and asked me: 'I am allowed to eat pigeon soup every now and then, aren't I?' It was very difficult for him to stick to the diet. As soon as his physician told him his condition had improved, he stopped following the diet. Nevertheless he referred other cancer patients to me. He must have known the diet had really helped him.

The First Step

The first step is the willingness to follow the diet and to apply it to the best of the patient's ability. The diet cannot be forced on anyone; people have to opt for it themselves. Very often relatives or friends come over to discuss the possibilities of the Dries diet with me. But as long as the patient him- or herself does not consult me, everything else is in vain. The diet may be recommended, but the first step towards the diet has to be made by the cancer patient him- or herself. There needs to be a positive attitude towards the diet and towards nutritional therapy in general. Patients need to devote all their energies to it, and to be convinced that this therapy is useful and that it is very important in order to support the recovery process. If patients dawdle over their food or if they are not fully convinced of the value of the diet, there's no point in applying it.

A look at the seven groups of foodstuffs will immediately show that fruit is very important. The diet consists of two fruit meals complemented by a vegetable meal. The vegetable meal can be replaced regularly by a fruit meal. A very common reaction of cancer patients, relatives or neighbours is: 'Man cannot live on fruit alone!' That reaction is understandable in light of the fact that in traditional dietetics fruit is always considered a snack or dessert. In traditional dietetics fruit has always been neglected because of its low calorific value. But lately that has changed; fruit is now looked upon as a source of vitamins and minerals. But still fruit is not considered to be sustaining food. We will prove that the Dries diet complies with all nutritional standards and that shortages of any kind are not possible. The Dries diet offers the dieter so much more than ordinary, industrialized food. It is a big mistake to remain under the illusion that traditional food is ideal. Traditional food can be strongly criticized.

Humans are frugivores by nature. A comparison between the human digestive system and those of other frugivores makes this clear. Therefore the diet allows humans to start eating their original foodstuffs again. This means that those who are following the diet are in fact eating the food their digestive systems are made for. Our entire metabolism is tuned in to fruit. Humankind has eaten agricultural products for centuries and should know by now that those products lead to difficult and painful digestion. The Dries diet is easily digestible. It results in perfect digestion and efficient metabolism. Even though no great amounts are to be eaten, the dieter manages to get a lot out of the food.

An Algerian physician working as a neurosurgeon in Germany

came to visit me because he could not believe I had helped one of his patients simply by applying the diet. At first his patient had only little chance of survival, but now she is very healthy. He concluded the following: the body uses little energy to digest the food prescribed by the diet and to convert it into energy. Because of that, there is enough energy left to fight the disease. I have often thought about this statement. It is indeed a fact – I have read several books about this – that it takes an enormous amount of energy to digest ordinary food. Meat, fish, cheese, grain products and pulses are all very difficult to digest. A ripe peach, a banana, a kiwi or a mango, on the other hand, just melts in your mouth; this means that the precious sugars are absorbed immediately.

I believe that fruit has to be our basic food as fruit contains everything we need. Some of my patients ate solely foodstuffs from Group I. They did not starve; their weight remained stable; there were no shortages, as was proven by blood analysis. And all of them improved. Of course, people who are used to a well-laden table need to adjust a little bit. But after a while, everyone becomes convinced of the fact that traditional dietetics is in need of urgent amendments. A number of established opinions on the subject of foodstuffs seem to be wrong.

Now to discuss the components of the Dries diet. For the aspects of food I cannot find space to discuss here, I refer the reader to my other books.

Calories

It is only logical that the diet is low-calorie, because it consists mainly of watery fruits. The Dries diet is completely different from many popular diets based on the use of calories. Nutrients (proteins, fats and carbohydrates) are converted into energy. When people exert themselves physically, they burn calories, when practising a sport, they need more energy than when not exerting themselves. Even when at rest, the body needs heat-energy to make all the bodily functions possible. The most common question is: 'Won't we have a shortage of calories if we follow the diet?' The answer is no. Because everything is eaten raw. according to nutritional rules, the diet makes sure that digestion is optimal and metabolism is efficient. This means that – even though the dieter will burn fewer calories – he or she will get more out of them. In eating traditional food, between 2,000 and 3,000 Kcal a day are used because many foodstuffs are not or are only partially digested. There is a loss of calories, which leads to pollution of the body. With the Dries diet, the calorie supply is equal to consumption, so that there is no loss, nor pollution. The dieter should not start calculating the amount of calories in the food, though: it will only cause confusion. Cancer patients who manage to make do with only little food obtain very good results. Their weight remains stable; they can handle all kinds of exertion; they are not hungry and they feel well. It is obvious that they do not have a calorie shortage. If that is not the case, it is always possible to increase the amount of high-calorie foodstuffs. Examples of high-calorie foodstuffs are: almonds, nuts, seeds, avocados, whipped cream, oil dressings, mayonnaise and cottage cheese. It is no problem to reach 2,000Kcal a day with this diet, but if the dieter can make do with less (and most of the time that is the case), that is a lot better.

Proteins

If a patient asks a physician whether he or she objects to the Dries diet, the physician will possibly answer: 'It doesn't look bad, but make sure you get enough proteins.' Some physicians are very resolute and will immediately claim the diet cannot provide the patient with the necessary proteins. Proteins are at the centre of dietetics. The word 'protein' is derived from Greek and means 'the most important'. Protein is indeed the most important nutrient, but that does not necessarily mean we need large quantities of it. Traditional dietetics is only interested in the amount and the biological value of protein. Biological value is determined by means of the essential amino acids at hand: amino acids are the components of protein. In traditional dietetics, most proteins are characterized by a poor biological value: the proteins are nearly always damaged as a result of preparation techniques. They are difficult to digest because the food combinations are not taken into account. People eat everything at random. Too much protein and especially badly digested protein leads to an enormous pollution and acidification of the tissues. Many scientists are convinced that a tumour feeds on protein residues and that every diet should be low protein. Scientific research has shown that the human needs only ½oz (15g) of protein a day, as long as that amount contains all the necessary amino acids. That also means the protein supply has to be replenished every day. Fruit contains very little protein (an average of 1 per cent), but if a person eats 2.2lb (1kg) of fruit a day, he or she already has ⅓oz (10g) of protein of a very high biological quality. If 2oz (60g) of almonds are added to that (18 per cent protein) and 17½oz (500g) of vegetables (2 per cent protein), a total of 2oz (30g) of protein will be reached. That is double the amount needed per day. Patients who take yoghurt, cottage cheese, buttermilk, sunflower seeds, sesame seed, avocados, and other high-protein foodstuffs will easily reach 2–2½oz (60–70g) a day, but that is really too much. The World Health Organization (WHO) recommends 0.75g of protein for each kg of body weight. This means that a person who weighs 132lb (60kg) needs 1⅝oz (45g) of protein a day, and that someone who weighs 176lb (80kg) needs about 2oz (60g) of protein a day. These standards are very easy to reach but the question is whether that is the most sensible thing to do. Especially in the case of cancer it is extremely important not to exceed the real need for protein. We are more concerned about an excess than we are about a shortage. People who follow a diet that mainly consists of fruit, supplemented with 1¾oz (50g) of almonds or other nuts, do not suffer from a protein shortage. Cancer patients have to undergo a blood analysis regularly. Not one of my patients has ever been diagnosed with a protein shortage. With my diet, the need for protein is much lower than with other diets. The Dries diet makes sure you have a much better protein metabolism and that has a significant influence on the recovery process.

This table clearly shows the very good composition of the fruit-protein. 1kg of fruit produces 7–11g of protein. 100g of almonds produces 16g of protein. All this is high-quality protein. The amino acids in bold are the essential amino acids.

Fats

When I ask people whether they watch what they eat, they nearly always tell me: 'We don't use much fat.' Low-fat food

	Mango	Avocado	Guava	Persimmon	Neffel
Alanine	-	7,5	7,5	7,7	6,4
Arginine	4,6	2,9	3,9	3,4	3,7
Asparagine acid	9,3	10,9	9.7	13,9	12,1
Cystine	0,9	0,3	-	0,8	0,3
Glutamine acid	13,3	13,1	-	10,1	17,2
Glycine	4,9	6,5	7,5	6,5	6,0
Histidine	**3,0**	**1,5**	**1,2**	**2,3**	**1,3**
Isoleucine	**4,6**	**5,1**	-	**5,1**	**4,4**
Leucine	**7,5**	**8.9**	-	**9,9**	**7,1**
Lysine	**6,6**	**7,5**	**5,8**	**7,5**	**6,2**
Methionine	**1,7**	**2,0**	**0,8**	**1,0**	**1,2**
Fenyalanine	**4,4**	**5,2**	**3,7**	**5,4**	**3,8**
Proline	4,6	5,1	4,6	5,7	-
Serine	4,9	5,4	4,5	5,1	6,2
Threonine	**4,6**	**5,3**	-	**5,1**	**4.0**
Tyrosine	2,5	3,5	-	3,9	2,9
Valine	**6,8**	**7,7**	**5,3**	**7,1**	**6,4**

Figure 10 *Amino acids in fruits, in terms of g/100g*

always seems to be taken as synonymous with healthy food. Nothing is further from the truth. The entire theory regarding food fats and health is a fabrication spread by margarine manufacturers. After thirty years of discussing saturated, unsaturated and polyunsaturated fatty acids, we have only now come to the conclusion that heated polyunsaturated fatty acids are the greatest enemy for our health. They make it possible for free radicals to develop and free radicals are considered carcinogenic.

All the fats in the Dries diet are used unheated. Almonds, nuts, seeds and avocados produce fats in their most natural form. Extra fat is only used when you add whipped cream or cold-pressed oil (an oil dressing), vinaigrette or mayonnaise to the vegetables. Fat has a number of good qualities and does not have to be avoided. Basically, the Dries diet is cholesterol-free. Egg yolk, curd cheese and yoghurt are the only components of the diet that contain a small amount of cholesterol, but that amount is negligible.

Carbohydrates

In dietetics, 'carbohydrates' is the collective name for sugars. There are various kinds of sugar, but the most important ones are the simple, double and complex sugars. The complex sugars are more commonly known as 'starch'. By nature, the human metabolism is only capable of absorbing simple sugars, which means that double and complex sugars have to be decomposed first. The decomposition process involves a high energy consumption and several auxiliary substances such as vitamins and minerals. In traditional food, starch is very important. Agricultural products – such as grains, pulses and root crops – produce large amounts of starch. Most people eat high-starch food.

The Dries diet is starch-free and that has some clear advantages. It smoothens digestion and metabolism; the dieter will save not only on energy, but also on vitamins and minerals. Once his or her digestive system is adjusted to the starch-free diet, the dieter will be able to benefit from all the advantages mentioned in this book. Your blood sugar level will tune in to the supply of simple sugars and will remain very stable because of that. Unfortunately there are cancer patients who can't do without starch. They keep on losing weight and are not able to reach their ideal weight. These patients are temporarily forced to use small amounts of starch until their body weight stabilizes. Sugars are not only quantitatively but also qualitatively the most important nutrients in the fight against cancer. The Dries diet contains lots of unrefined, simple sugars (that is, sugars that are naturally occurring parts of foodstuffs).

Water

There are several watery foodstuffs in the Dries diet. Most foodstuffs in the diet – with the exception of nuts and seeds – contain a lot of water. Water is the most important substance in the body and good water regulation is the key to health. Watery foodstuffs are easy to digest. They provide a good acid-base balance, which rules out acidification. To obtain a favourable acid-base balance, we should eat good amounts of watery foodstuffs that also contain a large amount of metals (min. 80 per cent), and we should eat only small amounts (max. 20 per cent) of concentrated foodstuffs. After all, concentrated foodstuffs contain much less water and are full of non-metals. During metabolism, non-metals are converted into acids that are eliminated by means of the buffer systems (blood, kidneys and respiration). If there are any superfluous acids, they are stored in the tissues, which leads to a disruption of the mineral regulation (demineralization) and a general pollution of the entire organism. Some people call this acidification the food for the tumour.

Vitamins

The Dries diet undoubtedly contains a lot of vitamins. Vitamins are bio-catalysts that make bio-chemical processes possible. On their own, vitamins do not have any value, but together with the nutrients to which they are linked, they do. Vitamins are very vulnerable substances. Freezing or conserving foodstuffs results in a loss of vitamins. Preparing foodstuffs is synonymous to destroying vitamins, either partially or completely, especially when the preparation takes place at a high temperature. In raw food, however, the vitamins remain intact, and bear a proper proportion to the nutrients. If you suffer from a shortage of certain vitamins, you can replenish that shortage by using foodstuffs that contain a good amount of vitamins. Generally, the amount of vitamins in this diet is a lot higher than traditional dietetics requires. The use of vitamin preparations and multivitamins is no good at all. They pollute the organism. A vitamin preparation cannot be compared to a nutritional vitamin. (See my discussion of food supplements, pp. 102–3.)

Minerals

The same can be said about minerals and trace elements (micronutrients). On their own, these substances are not important either, but they also are significant in proportion to the nutrients. People think that minerals can withstand heat better, but that is not true. The cooking or baking temperature renders minerals inactive. The electromagnetic field that is very important to minerals (because it makes their catalytic action possible) disappears when you heat them. Inactive minerals have a disturbing effect on the kidney filters, which have to make sure they are removed. People and animals have to rely on food for their supply of minerals; only plants are capable of absorbing minerals directly from the earth's surface and converting them into active minerals during photosynthesis. We do not recommend the use of mineral preparations because they consist of inactive minerals, which burden the organism.

Sodium–Potassium proportion

Books about nutrition will mention the importance of sodium and potassium, but often overlook the fact that it is the proportion of sodium to potassium that is extremely important. By using salt as a flavouring or a preservative, we completely disrupt the sodium–potassium proportion. Natural food contains only small amounts of sodium, as opposed to a great deal of potassium – in a banana, the proportion is 1/380. Tinned food-stuffs and other industrial foodstuffs contain more sodium than potassium. The Dries diet contains a large amount of potassium and only a small amount of sodium, resulting in an intense water secretion, which relieves the heart. After all, potassium is heart-friendly. According to some researchers, the sodium–potassium proportion in the cells plays an important part in the fight against cancer. Cancer patients whose kidneys do not function properly or who only have one kidney, should be cautious, however: the kidneys should have enough eliminating capacity to meet the water-secreting effect of the potassium. If that is not the case, the diet needs to be adjusted. When in doubt, such patients should consult a kidney specialist.

Free radicals

We have already mentioned how dangerous heated fats are. Heating fats result in the development of lipidperoxides, which not only affect the vascular walls of the cells, but also the DNA. If any essential molecules are affected, there is a possibility that cancer will develop. Smoked fish, ham, bacon, sausages, etc. are looked upon as carcinogenic in traditional dietetics, and so attempts are made to fight the development of free radicals by using antioxidants such as vitamin E, vitamin C, selenium, etc. The Dries diet does not entail any danger of free radicals. If a patient has too many free radicals, the diet will normalize them in no time.

Nitrate

Risks run through eating leaf vegetables are well known. Leaf vegetables have a very high nitrate content. Nitrate is converted into nitrite and nitride, which is converted into nitrosamine. Nitrosamine is a carcinogenic substance. What is often not known is that the conversion described here mainly takes place in meat. If we stick to eating vegetables, there is no danger at all. Furthermore, tomatoes contain cumarin and chlorogenes, both of which reduce the forming of nitrosamine.

Food supplements

Not only cancer patients but also other people think that the use of food supplements gets rid of all shortfall of necessary substances in one's diet. Unfortunately, they are mistaken. Food supplements are produced in laboratories and contain a large number of substances such as vitamins, minerals and amino acids. But it would be too convenient if we could replenish all shortfall with bottled substances. These expensive products are widely advertised, even though there is no proof of their effects. Indeed, that is not a requirement, because they are not considered medication. Prof. Dr Peter Schauder of the University of Göttingen (Germany) says: 'A one-sided approach to only a single nutrient is problematic, because the various macro- and micronutrients influence each other and are able to strengthen or weaken each other during bio-chemical processes.'[1] Moreover, a

[1] Peter Schauder, *Ernährung und Tumorenkrankungen*, Karger, Basel, 1991, p. 4.

distinction has to be made between a vitamin (or mineral) that is part of a living organism, and a vitamin (or mineral) that is part of a tablet or capsule. Bio-energetic research has unsettled the credibility of food supplements. Only natural food supplements contain substances that are accepted by the cells. All other substances are rejected or lead to pollution of the body. Much of the research done in the last few years indicates that frequent use of carotene stimulates the development of lung cancer in smokers. The use of megadoses of vitamin C in the form of a preparation annuls the positive effects of selenium. All this research suggests that preparations do more harm than good. I hope it will soon become clear that preparations lead only to bodily pollution. Just because people think a preparation can replenish all shortfall, they are all too ready to dose themselves with it.

One cancer patient told me that he had to take 24 tablets each day for a whole year; the tablets consisted of vitamins, minerals and other substances. When he showed me the leaflet that recommended the tablets, I understood why he really believed in them. In the leaflet I read: 'Nothing in nature contains so many active substances at the same time.' But the patient insisted he had not noticed any improvement – the cancer had just developed normally. Food supplements are polluting; they are unnatural and completely in defiance of the basic principles of natural medicine and dietetics. But a distinction should be made between food supplements and biological preparations that are considered natural medication. There are a number of quite food preparations for the treatment of cancer which have a favourable influence on the body's defence mechanism.

The Switchover

The Dries diet is very attractive, tastes good, gives a pleasant feeling in stomach and bowels, is easily digestible and produces repletion rapidly. Nobody starves when following this diet. Only the sudden switchover to the diet is sometimes rather un-expected. People who suffer from other illnesses can switch over to another diet very slowly, so that their digestive systems can get used to it. But cancer patients lack the time to do so, which is why many cancer patients switch over to the diet the same day they come to see me. That sudden switchover is not only a physical but also an emotional strain. Patients later tell me: 'The first week I went through hell.' But what can be expected with so little time to adjust? One cancer patient who had already been applying my nutritional principles for years, and who had already changed his diet drastically years ago, told me he still had trouble switching over to the strict diet. He also told me: 'I can imagine that people who are not familiar with natural food have a lot of trouble switching over to the diet.' I do not want to disguise the truth: the patient has to get used to the diet. Many people have been sitting at tables full of steaming dishes, stacks of sandwiches, huge pieces of meat and all kinds of spicy or salted food all their lives, and then suddenly they have to make do with a slice of pineapple, half a kiwi and a piece of mango. Many people find comfort in the fact that they are allowed to put some whipped cream or yoghurt on top of their food. Still, not everyone is enthusiastic about the diet, even knowing that it will help them. Dr Nolfi once said: 'The day I discovered I had cancer and had to face death – a painful death within about two years – it was not difficult for me to switch over to a raw food diet. I was grateful that something as simple as that could help me.' That is how most patients look at it. They are glad that there is a balanced diet that significantly increases their chances of recovery and that relieves the side-effects of the heavy, regular treatment. That is why they switch over so soon. Most people experience scarcely any problems when they do that: everything goes well right from the start. A physician who had started following the diet himself told me (much to my surprise): 'Now I eat everything I never used to eat before.' When they diagnosed him with cancer for the second time, they told me he had little chance of recovery. He started following the diet because he had no other option, and against all odds he recovered in no time.

Many people still go on for a long time craving hot potatoes, generously filled sandwiches, fried eggs or cheese. But everyone completely agrees that such food cannot possibly be part of the diet. The need for meat or fish reduces quite quickly: it does not take long for someone to get used to a meatless diet. By eating everything raw, the dieter cleanses the entire organism. Cooked food, however small the amount may be, disrupts the important cleansing process. The cleaner the food, the more bio-energy is stored. Cooked food is characterized by disrupted bio-energy, which means that the body has to repair that bio-energy in order to make part of the food useful again. That implies an enormous loss of the energy that should have been used in the recovery process.

In exceptional cases, there are people who cannot keep to the diet. They have trouble adjusting to the food and try to find all kinds of compromises. They eat the prescribed food, but they add a sandwich or one hot meal a day to it. That is not a solution, though, the diet has to be followed very strictly. If the patient refuses to open his or her mind to the diet and merely considers it an obligation, there is no point in following the diet. The digestive system is triggered by a craving for food; if a person has an aversion to the food he or she is eating, or is reluctant to eat it, he or she blocks the hunger centre, which will make the stomach close. From this it may be concluded that the psychological aspect of nutritional therapy is very important. An example: if someone is just about to eat and receives an unpleasant phone call, it can spoil the appetite.

Whoever has a positive attitude towards the diet will be able to forget old eating habits much easier. Many patients say: 'This food tastes wonderful.' They discover the aroma of natural food and are able to enjoy it. After a week it is as if they have always eaten this kind of food. Some women tell me it is very easy for them to stay away from the food they cook for their families every day. And one of my former patients continued applying the diet after she had been declared completely cured. She liked the diet so much that nothing in the world could make her go back to her old eating habits. The foodstuffs used in the Dries diet are delicious, but the ideas that have been programmed into our brains make us think differently about that. Someone who quits smoking permanently, stops craving nicotine. My family and I have been leading a vegetarian life for twenty-five years now, and it's no hardship at all.

We advice everyone to switch over to the diet gradually during the first week, so that its full application can be started during the second week. During the first week, old eating habits have to be run down, one day at a time. That way some of the old eating habits can be replaced by a part of the new diet every day. For example, drinking coffee can be reduced in order to create a completely 'coffee-free' state after six days. The same can be done with meat, cheese, bread and other foodstuffs. As can be seen, the switchover does not have to be complicated. All one has to do is to start with one fruit meal a day and then to take two fruit meals a day. Meanwhile, use of traditional food gradually stops. Sticking to the following chart will help:

1 First day: One fruit meal
2 Second day: Two fruit meals
3 Third day: Two fruit meals
4 Fourth day: Two fruit meals
5 Fifth day: Two fruit meals and a vegetable meal
6 Sixth day: Two fruit meals and a vegetable meal

Of course, eating some fruit or drinking some freshly squeezed orange juice is allowed between meals. Some people want to switch over to the diet from the first day on. I usually recommend against doing that, because both body and mind need time to adjust to the diet. To be able to run down one's old habits and to switch over to the diet in six days is already a great accomplishment.

Reactions

Usually there are certain reactions, but they are quite normal and need not be cause for worry. Possible reactions are:

- Urinating more and also more often because of the large amount of potassium
- tendency towards diarrhoea, because of bowels are over-stimulated by the fruit fibres
- constipation in spite of the large amounts of fruit
- rash as a result of purification
- dizziness, nervousness or fatigue because the detoxification process is too slow
- temporary insomnia
- temporary weight loss
- coated tongue and bad breath
- smelly stools
- increased flatulence
- feeling of repletion fails to occur
- shivering
- sensitivity to cold, especially when the patient starts following the diet during the winter
- stomach and/or intestinal complaints if the patient cannot tolerate raw vegetables

Once again: it must be stressed that these reactions are no cause for concern. They have to do with adjustment to the diet and purification of the body. They will disappear spontaneously as soon as digestion and metabolism have adjusted completely. Initially the dieter might eat large quantities of food under the impression that he or she cannot get a feeling of satiation. That impression gradually fades though. Once the digestive system had adjusted, the digestion of nutrients takes place in a normal way. Body weight, which has decreased during the switchover, becomes stable again: this stabilization is often the turning point in the recovery process. From that moment on, the dieter will start to feel better. It is good not only to urinate more but also to urinate more often, which will be the case for as long as the patient applies the diet; excessive urinating occurs very seldom and is usually caused by something else. People with a kidney malfunction are usually not capable of processing large amounts of potassium, which is why they have to start by adding a small amount of fruit to each meal, and they can later gradually increase the amount of fruit. When in doubt, they should contact their GP or a kidney specialist.

In case of persistent diarrhoea, the best thing to do is to drink diluted bilberry juice and to gradually decrease the amount of fruit per meal until the intestines function properly again. In case of constipation, 'colon clean', a natural cure based on fenugreek seed can be used. If a rash develops, help can come from use of a purifying tea of which you can find the recipe further on in this chapter (p. 145). In case of slow detoxication, it is important for the dieter to treat him- or herself to warm baths and to exercise as much as possible. As well, a herb tea composed of equal parts of elderberry blossoms, lime blossoms and marigold can be used. If the dieter has the shivers, he or she should exercise; if sensitive to cold, he or she should dress warmly and make sure to get enough exercise; if experiencing stomach complaints or intestinal complaints after having eaten raw vegetables, he or she should liquidize the vegetables in a blender and – if necessary – replace the vegetable meal with a fruit meal. After a few weeks all these reactions will have disappeared and his or her digestive system will function better than it has ever done before. The dieter must not let temporary adjustment problems be any cause for alarm.

Losing weight

Switching over to this diet is not the only cause of weight loss. When someone suspects he or she has cancer and especially when the suspicion is confirmed, the shock is so tremendous that he or she can start to lose weight spontaneously. Waiting for the results of the examination can almost always be accomplished by a lack of appetite. The stomach cuts itself off from tensions, which is one reason why the patient becomes unable to eat. Because cancer patients can frequently be of the slender type, their weight loss catches the eye sooner. The hospitalization, the surgery and of course the radiation therapy or chemotherapy can play havoc with the patient's appetite. That is how weight loss can develop.

When cancer patients start with the diet early on in the therapy, we can still do something about weight loss, but much of the time they have already gone through part of the treatment. In that case they have already lost a lot of weight and the last thing they want to hear is that they are going to lose some more. This needs to be expected if the digestive system has to process food that it has to get used to. Some patients only lose a couple of kilos, but sometimes the weight loss is considerable. In any case, the patient's weight is carefully checked and kept up to date. The weight loss may also be a consequence of the regular treatment and sometimes the weight loss develops because the disease continues to develop or because the patient is unable to retain enough fluids. Such patients have a hard time adjusting to a starch-free diet. After all, one of the properties of starch is that it retains fluids. In such cases we are forced to add some foodstuffs that contain starch to the diet, at least until the weight stabilizes. Once the patient has switched over to the diet, his or her weight becomes stable again, even if the quantity of food is reduced. Cancer patients who follow the diet come to us every four weeks so that we can discuss their condition and so that we can adapt their diet if necessary. Many cancer patients suffer from anorexia or from malnutrition as a consequence of the severe treatments. It is obvious that such patients cannot start with the Dries diet immediately. The best thing for them to do is to normalize their weight first; during that process both the emotional aspect and the quality of their digestive system play an important part.

Raw vegetables

It is evident that no one is bothered by the use of fruit; but there are often complaints about problems with raw vegetables. Those problems can be rather serious for some people. That depends on the quality of their digestive systems. Humans are not herbivores by nature and raw vegetables can be quite fibrous. If there are problems with raw vegetables, the best thing to do is to purée the vegetables, liquidize them or limit the quantity of vegetables in the diet. As has been noted of the foodstuffs in each of the seven groups, vegetables are less important in this diet. If a patient is really bothered by the vegetables, he or she can switch over to three fruit meals a day. Vegetables are not absolutely necessary, but they are part of the diet because many people appreciate a raw vegetable dish with a scrumptious dressing. That is especially important if there are problems in switching over to sweet foods. With the Dries diet, we intend to have the patients switch over to things with a sweet taste. Their taste has to be depolarized – that is, they have to develop a taste for sweet things in order to replace their taste for sour–salty things. Patients who do not succeed in doing that will not be able to obtain results with this diet.

Fruit

Fruit has to be very ripe and preferably of biological quality. If possible, fruit should be ripened after it has been picked and before being eaten. It should be sliced with a sharp knife and eaten piece by piece. Small pieces of fruit should be left to melt in the mouth, because that is the best way to eat fruit. Most people eat fruit far too quickly, and that is why they eat too much of it. If fruit is eaten slowly, the sugars in the fruit are released slowly and will influence the saturation centre. There will be a feeling of repletion in no time. But if, on the other hand, fruit is eaten too quickly, the saturation centre will only respond when the stomach expands, which impels one to eat large quantities. The stomach cannot deal with such large quantities, and there will be fermentation. I know of people who eat very large quantities of fruit and who still do not feel satisfied. Those who follow the diet are expected to eat small quantities of bio-energetically beneficial food so that their body weight remains stable or increases slightly; that means they have perfect digestion. It is not the quantity of food on the plate that is important, but the amount of nutrients the digestive system can get out of it.

Sensitivity to cold

If following the diet starts during autumn or winter, there will probably be some sensitivity to cold, especially during the first period; that is because the dieter's thermoregulation needs some time to adjust. Most patients have been using steaming hot dishes for years and that way they have brought large amounts of artificial heat into their bodies. Food has to reach body temperature before it can be digested. If we eat warm food, our internal thermostat reacts by shutting off the heat supply, so that the food can cool down. What happens if we suddenly start eating raw food? The temperature of raw food is lower than our body temperature, which means that our body has to heat up the cold food until it reaches body temperature. That process uses up body heat, which is why sensitivity to cold can sometimes last for hours and hours. Our body is made for digesting cold food and has more trouble digesting warm food. That is why we usually feel tired after having eaten a warm meal. Sensitivity to cold is a normal reaction that disappears after a while.

If body heat drains away too quickly when raw food is being eaten, the dieter will start shivering. The best way to get rid of shivering is to move about (exercise), to rest under a woollen blanket or to move closer to a heat source. Some people even suffer from sensitivity to cold and shivering during the summer, especially if they are predisposed to doing so. In the beginning, the lack of calories in the diet may also be responsible for sensitivity to cold, because not enough calories are released. That is one of the reasons why we recommend a gradual switchover.

People who are following a treatment that implies fasting are not allowed to eat anything. Because they cannot build up a heat supply with regard to food calories, their body cools down considerably. That drop in temperature only takes place on the outside of the body, though; the internal temperature remains quite stable. Initially these people experience a weird feeling, as if they have turned into stone.

On the other hand, food should not be too cold either, especially not on cold days. The best thing to do is to make sure the foodstuffs are at room temperature. If shivering or sensitivity to cold are really bothersome, the food can be placed on a radiator or heated in the oven (*not* in a microwave, which changes the molecular structure of the foodstuffs, and use of which is strictly forbidden by our diet). So that the quality of the food does not suffer, it should only be heated to a maximum of 40°C. Some patients, however, have a great need for warm food. Those patients can drink warm herb tea and eat warm raw soup, but all the rest has to be cold. During a hot summer none of these problems is likely to occur.

Stomach- and intestinal problems

If the diet causes stomach- or intestinal problems, it means you have been eating too large quantities of raw vegetables. The stomach cannot process large quantities of food. If the dieter has stomach- and intestinal problems, the best thing to do is to stop eating vegetables. Fast for a few days. Drink a suitable herb tea (aniseed, fennel seed, camomile or lavender blossom) during those days. Switch over to fruit as much as possible.

Aphthae

People with aphthae are often told they should not eat pineapples because the mucous membranes of the mouth become too irritated. That can be the result of chemotherapy or of a thorough purging of the body. What can be done about it? Rinsing the mouth with camomile tea that contains honey (1–2 tsp (5–10ml) per cup) will help. Both camomile and honey are extremely efficient against infections. And to eat pineapple, squeeze it and drink the juice with a straw; a little bit of whipped cream or rich yoghurt may be added to it. This emulsifies the acid so that it loses its aggressive effects.

Drinking for Good Health

In recent years, it has frequently been claimed that we have to drink 3–5 pints (2–3 litres) of water a day in order to stay healthy. That statement is not based on anything official or significant. People who drink a lot of coffee, eat a lot of salted meat, eat a lot of grain products or other unhealthy food probably should drink a lot. That way they can at least wash down part of the toxic substances. But there is only one sensible rule: we should drink when thirsty. Some people have a greater need for drinking than others. Because the Dries diet mainly consists of watery foodstuffs, those who follow this diet have a lesser need to drink. Eliminating coffee and alcohol makes that need decrease also. Drinking spring water, fruit- or vegetable juice and herb tea is permitted. Herb tea may be drunk hot or cold. Substitute coffees are not allowed because they consist of burnt substances. For people who are healthy, using substitute coffees is a good way of getting rid of their addiction to coffee. But substitute coffees do not belong in this diet. Alcoholic beverages such as wine and beer are forbidden, because alcohol hampers the absorption of minerals and vitamins as well as possessing other unfavourable properties. Non-alcoholic beer may be drunk once in a while, but certainly not every day.

Fruit juice as liquid food

Of course drinking fresh-squeezed fruit juice is permitted in the diet. Fruit juice has the advantage of being a liquid and can be compared to mother's milk. It is very easily digestible and is generally absorbed without any problems. It is important to drink fruit juice very slowly. Too often, fruit juice is drunk too quickly and in too-large quantities. There is no reason not to introduce a juice day or to take a juice cure of several days, as long as all the juice is not drunk in one go. Just as a baby drinks its mother's milk in small quantities, juice should be taken one sip at a time. Some very ill patients who could no longer eat solids have been able to achieve very good results by doing this. Each time they were administered only one tablespoon (15ml) of juice, for example, every 15 minutes.

It must be taken into account that squeezing fruit or vegetables involves an enormous loss of energy. There is a very big difference between the nutrients of a pineapple or an orange and those of the juices. Squeezing a fruit and only using its juice utilizes only a small part of it. A volume of 3½fl oz of juice of a certain foodstuff nearly always contains fewer nutrients than the same quantity of the same foodstuff. When a pineapple is squeezed, for example, there will be obtained only as many nutrients as half a pineapple would provide. Juice has to be squeezed fresh daily. If not, its bio-energetic value will drop considerably as a result of too much oxidation. But that does not alter the fact that juice is valuable and may certainly be used. Beware of juice cures that call for drinking more than 9 pints (5 litres) of juice every day, though; if there is real need to drink large quantities of juice, it should be done under professional supervision.

Following the Dries Diet

We have discussed the diet elaborately and we have paid a considerable amount of attention to the switchover. Furthermore, we have discussed a number of possible reactions and problems. With that knowledge at the back of our minds, we will now describe the various possibilities for following the diet.

Initially, most people eat more vegetables than fruit, because vegetables are closer to ordinary food, but eventually discover the wonderful flavour of fruit, the better digestion and the feeling of repletion it brings. As much fruit as desired can be eaten – the dieter is certainly not supposed to starve. But it is wrong to think that large quantities are needed in order to promote recovery. Smaller amounts of fruit can be digested more easily, which means more can be got out of it. Everyone is free to determine how much he or she wants to eat each day, but the quantity of food should be determined spontaneously, and not with the help of scales. It is up to the dieter to decide. If he or she prefers not to eat a certain foodstuff, there is no pressure to eat it. If a certain foodstuff cannot be tolerated or if there is an aversion to it, that foodstuff is not suitable for use. But because many foodstuffs of the Dries diet are unknown to the dieter, he or she has to learn to eat some of them. There are people who don't like avocado at first. Those people often have problems with their gall bladder, which complicates the digestion of fats. What they should do is to cut the avocado in half, take out the stone and add a fair amount of lemon juice to the flesh. Then they will be able to enjoy the avocado. The lemon juice emulsifies the fat and makes it easier to digest. Moreover, the lemon juice gets rid of the dull, fatty taste completely. Some people cannot appreciate the turpentine aroma of the mango, until they have acquired a taste for it. Some time must be taken to adjust to these new flavours.

The first group

The first group consists of the foodstuffs with the highest bio-energetic values. If the condition of the patient is serious, we compose the diet solely with foodstuffs of the first group. But we do add almonds to the diet, in order to cover the need for protein. It has already been mentioned that some whipped cream can be added to the fruit, not only to make the fruit meals a little bit more tasty, but also to improve digestion. One of the properties of fat is that it slows down digestion, which allows the food to stay in the stomach longer. Better digestion means a better absorption of the nutrients.

A diet that consists solely of the foodstuffs of the first group can be followed for several months, as long as almonds are added to it. That way the diet contains all the necessary nutrients. An alternative is to follow a diet that consists of foodstuffs of the seven groups and regularly switch over to foodstuffs of the first group for a few days or a full week. We have been able to reach surprising results with these diets. One of my female patients had a brain tumour that was not operable because its location was inaccessible. It was claimed that she had no chance of recovery. After she had followed the Dries diet very strictly for two months, it was discovered that the tumour had disappeared. All treatments were discontinued. Another patient who found himself in a similar situation followed the daily menus that are based on the seven groups. His diet was not that strict. After three months his tumour also had disappeared completely. From this we may conclude that the results do not always depend on the strictness of the diet.

Pineapple

The first group consists of the foodstuffs with the highest bio-energetic values. Of those foodstuffs, pineapple is the most important. Most dieters consume one pineapple a day during the first three months, usually spreading it over two or three meals. The best are sun-ripened pineapples that have been imported by aeroplane. if they are not available at the supermarket, they can be ordered at most greengroceries; seven pineapples a week are needed. Simple gadgets can be had to help hollow out the heart of the pineapple and for slicing it.

Avocado

Avocados have to be eaten separately – that is, in between meals; but lemon juice should be added to them, as mentioned earlier. Avocados contain a lot of fat and 2 per cent of protein. They are very important fruits.

Almonds

Almonds belong to the second group, but they are essential in a diet that otherwise consists solely of foodstuffs of the first group. They should be soaked overnight in spring water, and drained the next morning; those needed immediately can be skinned, and the remaining soaked almonds can be used for the rest of that day. Use 1¾oz (50g) a day.

Pollen

Pollen is used in between meals. Pollen is a kind of miracle drug that gives great energy; 2–4tbsp (30–60ml) of pollen should be used each day. Only natural grains should be used – that is, no powders or tablets. Patients who are being treated with radiotherapy should use 6tbsp (90ml) a day; patients who are being treated with chemotherapy can also take that amount three or four days before the chemotherapy, since it will help them reduce the side-effects. The dry pollen can be put in the mouth and swallowed with a sip of herb tea, or it can be dissolved in either herb tea or yoghurt. If large amounts of pollen are used over a certain period of time, saturation may develop, spon-taneously giving the sensation that too much pollen is being used. In that case, its use should be suspended for a few weeks, and then started again with smaller amounts – for example, 2tbsp (30ml) a day. There are people who think that if pollen is so good, it cannot possibly be overused. That is not true though. It has already been mentioned that people who suffer from hay fever are often allergic to pollen; use of pollen is not suitable for them. It may increase their blood pressure, which is why people who suffer from hay fever and who use pollen regularly have to keep a close eye on their blood pressure. If it increases too much under the influence of pollen, they should decrease the amounts of pollen or omit pollen altogether.

Honeydew melon, raspberry and cactus fruits

These fruits are very seasonal and because of that they are not available throughout the entire year. They can be replaced with fruits of the second group that are available when any of these is not. But if a strict diet is being followed, use should be restricted to mainly the foodstuffs of the first group. See the chart on p. 147 for seasonal availability of the various fruits.

Comb honey

Comb honey is generally kept in square wooden trays in amounts of about 9oz (250g). Most dieters use one-sixth of a tray each evening; that is, about 1½–1¾oz (40–50g). The honey is sucked out of the comb and the wax taken out of the mouth: the wax is not eaten. Sometimes the structure of the wax is so delicate that there is nearly none left; inadvertently swallowed wax is removed through bowel movements. Comb honey is very sweet: after it is eaten, some herb tea can be drunk or used to rinse the mouth. Comb honey is generally used in the evening, because of its calming effect. Comb honey helps provide a good night's rest. The use of comb honey also prevents the development of aphthae, and if already present, they will disappear sooner. It is advisable to brush the teeth after taking comb honey because it sometimes leaves behind sugar residues which, on their own, are not dangerous; but they can be if the bacterial balance in the mouth is disrupted. Such disruption is usually the consequence of taking cooked food, in which case certain bacteria cause the sugar residues to be converted into aggressive acids which affect the dental enamel.

Monodiet

Following a monodiet means using only one single foodstuff for a certain period of time, usually 7–10 days. The advantage of a monodiet is that the digestive system has to process only one foodstuff, which is very easy. Besides which, certain foodstuffs have very good properties. If only one of those foodstuffs is used, its good properties can be exploited fully. Of course a monodiet is one-sided and cannot provide the full range of nutrients needed. That is why it must be applied over only a short period of time. Even though a monodiet is very useful in the fight against cancer, we have to take into account that a monodiet usually causes the body weight to drop. People who follow a monodiet always have a certain objective. A pineapple diet, for example, can have a strong influence on the metabolism. It can detoxify the entire organism and exercise a restraining influence on the tumour. A cherry cure, a persimmon cure or a mango cure can have the same effects – to a lesser degree, however.

If the patient suffers from water retention, monodiets that drain water can be a real blessing. Examples of monodiets that drain water include a banana cure, an orange cure, a watermelon cure, an apricot cure or even a milk cure (buttermilk cure). A monodiet is not important because of its energetic value; it should be looked upon instead as a support of the basic diet. A bilberry cure or a bilberry juice cure is ideal for people with intestinal problems and especially for people who suffer from persistent diarrhoea. If support is wanted for the liver because it is too weak or overburdened, or because it shows metastasis, a monodiet based on one of the following fruits may be followed: persimmon, kiwi, pineapple, apricot, bilberry or honeydew melon.

The Daily Menu

Most cancer patients choose their own daily menu – whatever they feel like, as long as it is available at the time. They do not have to use all the foodstuffs in the seven groups; it is advisable, though, that 40–50 per cent of the foodstuffs belong to group I and the rest of the foodstuffs to groups II and III. The foodstuffs of group IV, V, VI and VII must never dominate. They are complementary and should only represent 20 per cent of the daily menu. It is possible to eat more foodstuffs of groups I and II one day and eat more foodstuffs of groups III and IV the next day. That is no problem at all. The diet can be adapted to individual needs. We will now explain how to compose a daily menu.

On getting up:
Basically, the dieter starts the day with 1 or 2tbsp (15 or 30ml) of pollen either dry or dissolved in herb tea or juice. This is repeated during the evening (2–4tbsp (30–60ml) of pollen a day).
Breakfast:
The fruit breakfast consists of some fruits from groups I, II or III. (Pineapple must absolutely be part of the breakfast.) Some native fruits (groups IV and V) can also be added to the fruit breakfast. Whipped cream and yoghurt are allowed, but not necessary.

Mid-morning:

A minimum of 1¾oz (50g) of prepared almonds is to be used daily; the almonds can also be replaced with nuts or seeds mentioned in the various groups. The best thing to do is to divide the total amount into 2 × ¾oz (2 × 25g), more or less 2 × 15 almonds.

Midday meal:

Fresh, uncooked, home-made soup with fresh vegetables and vegetable stock (Vegemite) or vegetable pasta. Both of these seasonings contain quite a lot of salt and some cancer patients are worried about that; however, the amount of vegetable stock or vegetable pasta used in the uncooked soup is minimal, so that the soup contains only a limited amount of salt. The rest of the Dries diet is completely salt-free, but vegetables do contain natural sodium. If salt is not permitted because of a heart or kidney condition, it is clear that vegetable stock or vegetable pasta are also not allowed.

To the soup may be added 2tbsp (30ml) of wheat germ. The soup is prepared with warm water. Soup can also be consumed between meals or in the evening. This warm, raw soup gives the menu some variety and is appreciated by many cancer patients; there are several possible recipes – even avocado soup tastes wonderful.

The soup may be replaced with a starter; some examples of starters appear among the recipes for the daily menus.

The main course should be a raw vegetable dish with a tasty dressing or mayonnaise. Uncooked mushrooms should also be included. The vegetables used here belong to groups IV and V; also highly recommended are tomatoes, broccoli and cabbage because of their phytochemicals.

Teatime:

Examples can be found among the recipes for the daily menus. Teatime items correspond to these of the mid-morning snack. It does not matter whether the almonds are taken mid-morning or in the afternoon: it's all up to the dieter.

Evening meal:
A fruit meal, as in the morning.
At bedtime:
1½–2oz (40–50g) of comb honey with herb tea.

It is better to spread the total daily amount of food over five meals than to spread it over three. It is not an absolute necessity but it is better for the digestion. If the dieter works away from home the best thing to do is to take the fruit along and cut and eat it there. A fruit salad or fruit purée should not be taken along, because prepared fruit ferments very quickly. As mentioned earlier, the vegetable meal may be replaced with a fruit meal (three fruit meals a day) or vegetables may be taken in limited amounts.

Seven Menus

Inge Dries, author of *200 New Food Combining Recipes*, has composed seven daily menus to help everyone get started with the diet. Most people are really happy with these recipes, but they often observe: 'We can't cope with such amounts.' They do not have to. In the beginning, people always eat large quantities because they fear they will not get a feeling of having eaten enough. But once used to this new diet, the dieter will find his or her need for food dropping considerably. The order in which these daily menus are used is unimportant; these are just examples.

The weights and measures shown throughout the following lists and recipes are converted as shown below, with figures rounded to the nearest whole or fraction.

2.2 pounds (2.2lb)   = 35.2 ounces (35.2oz) = 1 kilogram (1kg)
1 ounce (1oz)   = 25g or 30 g (for
                                                convenience in
                                                conversions of small
                                                amounts)

1 fluid ounce (1fl oz)   · = 25 millilitres (25ml)
1 tablespoonful (1tbsp)   = 15 millilitres (15ml)
1 teaspoonful (1tsp)   = 5 millilitres (5ml)
1 cupful (1 cup)   = 8 fluid ounces (8fl oz) = 225ml
         and/or   =7 fluid ounces (7fl oz) = 200 ml (for
                                                   convenience as
                                                   above)

Day 1

Shopping list
1 large pineapple
1 kiwi
5oz (150g) of redcurrants or an apple
1 large avocado
1 lemon
1 small lettuce (you will only need to use ⅓ oz (10g) on Day 1)
⅓oz (10g) of watercress or garden cress
7oz (200g) of mushrooms
⅔oz (20g) of chervil
7oz (200g) of yoghurt
17½oz (500g) of strawberries
2 ripe pears
9oz (250g) of passion fruit (4)

- ON GETTING UP

1–2tbsp (15–30ml) of pollen

- BREAKFAST

Stuffed Pineapple

10½oz (300g) of ripe pineapple (½ pineapple)
3oz (80g) of kiwi
5oz (150g) of redcurrants or an apple
1oz (25g) of chopped hazelnuts

Cut the pineapple lengthwise. Remove the hard core and scoop out the flesh. Cut the flesh into cubes and put the cubes in a bowl. Peel the kiwi, slice it and add it to the pineapple cubes. Then add the rinsed currants or a grated apple (add lemon juice to the apple). Use the fruit salad to fill the hollow part of the pineapple and sprinkle the whole with the chopped hazelnuts.

• MID-MORNING

Pineapple Juice

10½ oz (300g) of pineapple (½ pineapple)

Use a liquidizer (blender) to squeeze the juice out of the pineapple.

• MIDDAY MEAL

To start:

Avocado Cocktail

5oz (150g) of avocado
⅓oz (10g) of lettuce
⅓oz (10g) of watercress or garden cress
lemon juice
if so desired a radish to garnish

Take a cocktail glass or a low ice-cream cup and fill it with the rinsed and shredded lettuce leaves. Peel the avocado and cut it into tiny cubes. Put the cubes on top of the lettuce and pour some lemon juice over the whole (sprinkle with optional herbs). Add a teaspoon of mayonnaise, garnish with watercress or garden cress and sprinkle with a tablespoon of wheat germ. (If a whole avocado seems too much, use half of it.)

Main course:

Mushroom–Chervil Salad

7oz (200g) of raw mushrooms
⅔oz (20g) of chervil
⅓oz (10g) of mustard (1 tsp)
⅔oz (20g) of safflower oil
⅙oz (5g) of garlic (1 clove)
⅓oz (10g) of lemon juice (2 tsp)
⅙oz (5g) of fresh parsley and basil.

Rub the mushrooms clean or peel them. Rinse the chervil, the parsley and the basil. Chop the herbs and add the mushroom slices. Mix the mustard, oil, lemon juice and (if so desired) some herbs in a bowl. Pour this dressing over the mushroom–chervil mixture, stir well and wait for one hour before serving it.

- TEATIME

Strawberry Yoghurt

7oz (200g) of yoghurt
7oz (200g) of strawberries
⅓oz (10g) of wheat germ
⅓oz (10g) of honey (1 tsp)

In a liquidizer (blender, mix the yoghurt with the rinsed strawberries. Pour the mixture into a tall glass and sprinkle it with wheat germ. Some honey may be used to sweeten it. If there are not any strawberries available, use another kind of fruit.

- EVENING MEAL

Stuffed Pear on a bed of Strawberries

10½oz (300g) of ripe pears
9oz (250g) of passion fruit (4)
10½oz (300g) of strawberries

Peel the pears and cut them in half, lengthwise. Use a small spoon to scoop out the cores, creating a hollow in each pear half. Fill the hollows with the flesh of the passion fruit. Rinse the strawberries and remove the stalks. Then slice the strawberries thinly and arrange the slices on a plate. Make sure they overlap one another. Arrange the stuffed pears on the bed of strawberries.

• BEFORE BEDTIME

1½–1¾oz (40–50g) of comb honey
herb tea

DAY 2

Shopping List
1 honeydew melon
7oz (200g) of raspberries or 1 kiwi
7oz (200g) of bilberries or 1 passion fruit
1 pineapple
1 cucumber
a few sprigs of chervil
a few sprigs of watercress
1 small lettuce or ⅓oz (10g) of lettuce from Day 1
⅔oz (20g) of mushrooms
8fl oz (200ml) of buttermilk
1 kiwi

• ON GETTING UP

1–2tbsp (15–30ml) of pollen

- BREAKFAST

Forest Fruits–Melon

17½oz (500g) of honeydew melon (1 melon)
3½oz (100g) of raspberries or 3oz (80g) of kiwi
3½oz (100g) of bilberries or 3½oz (100g) of passion fruit

Rinse the raspberries and bilberries and put them in a colander. Cut the melon in half and remove the seeds. Fill the melon halves with the fruits.

- MID-MORNING

Pineapple Juice

10½oz (300g) of pineapple (½ pineapple)

Use a liquidizer (blender) to squeeze the juice out of the pineapple.

- MIDDAY MEAL

To start:

Cold Cucumber Soup

7oz (200g) of cucumber (½ cucumber)
5¼oz (150g) of low-fat yoghurt
1 leaf of fresh peppermint
¼ clove of garlic
a few drops of lemon juice if so desired
chopped parsley

Peel the cucumber, de-seed and shred it. Add the yoghurt, the crushed garlic, and chopped peppermint leaf and (if so desired) the lemon juice. Mix the soup well and then refrigerate it for 1 to 2 hours. Garnish the soup with the parsley before serving it.

Main course:

Mixed Salad

⅓oz (10g) of lettuce
⅓oz (10g) of sesame seeds (1tsp (5ml))
5¼oz (150g) of tomatoes
⅔oz (20g) of mushrooms
⅙oz (5g) of watercress
oil dressing with herbs, based on 4 tsp (20ml) of safflower oil

Rinse and dry the lettuce leaves and arrange them on a plate. Sprinkle them with the sesame seeds. Rinse the tomatoes and cut them into pieces. Rub the mushrooms clean, slice them and arrange them on the salad bed, together with the tomatoes. Garnish the salad with watercress and serve it with an oil dressing. (See more about dressings later in this chapter.)

• TEATIME

Buttermilk

8fl oz (200ml) of buttermilk

Fill a glass with buttermilk and sprinkle it with wheat germ. The buttermilk may be sweetened with honey, maple syrup or sweet fruit if so desired.

• EVENING MEAL

Pineapple Cocktail

10½oz (300g) of pineapple (½ pineapple)
3½oz (100g) of raspberries
3½oz (100g) of bilberries
3oz (80g) of kiwi
whipped cream if so desired

Peel the pineapple, remove the hard core and the eyes and cut the flesh into bite-sized cubes. Rinse the fruits, remove the stalks carefully and mix the fruits with the pineapple cubes. Serve in a bowl or in glasses and add whipped cream if so desired.

• BEFORE BEDTIME

1½–1¾oz (40–50g) of comb honey
herb tea

Day 3

Shopping List
1 pineapple
10½oz (300g) of blue grapes
10½oz (300g) of mangos (2 mangos)
7oz (200g) of low-fat yoghurt
1 small oak leaf lettuce or other lettuce
⅓oz (10g) of watercress (1 punnet)
⅔oz (20g) of hazelnuts and brazil nuts
1 spear of chicory
⅔oz (20g) of chervil
1 apple
6 lychees

• ON GETTING UP

1–2tbsp (15–30ml) of pollen

• BREAKFAST

Pineapple on Cocktail Sticks
10½oz (300g) of pineapple (½ pineapple)
10½oz (300g) of grapes
¾oz (25g) of whipped cream

Cut the pineapple in half (breadthwise) and save one half for the evening meal. Peel the other half and cut the flesh into bite-size cubes. Rinse and dry the grapes and fasten them on the pineapple pieces with cocktail sticks or toothpicks. Pour the whipped cream in a bowl and serve it as a dip.

- MID-MORNING

Mango Yoghurt
5¼oz (150g) of mango

Purée half the mango and mix with yoghurt; sprinkle with wheat germ.

- MIDDAY MEAL

To start:

Raw Chervil Soup
⅔oz (20g) of chervil
10fl oz (250ml) of vegetable stock
optional herbs

Rinse the chervil, dry it and chop it finely. Heat the vegetable stock. Add the chervil and other herbs if so desired. Serve the soup immediately.

Main course:

Watercress Nest
⅓oz (10g) of oak leaf lettuce
⅔oz (20g) of watercress
¾oz (25g) of chopped hazelnuts and brazil nuts (1 tbsp (15ml))
3⅓oz (100g) of chicory
1tbsp (15ml) of mayonnaise
2tbsp (30ml) of low-fat yoghurt

½ clove of garlic
optional herbs

Rinse and dry the lettuce and the watercress. Arrange the lettuce in the middle of a pudding-plate and build a nest of watercress on top of it. Fill this nest with finely chopped chicory and sprinkle it with the chopped nuts. Use the remaining ingredients to make a dip and serve with the salad.

• TEATIME

Apple with Hazelnuts

5¼oz (150g) of apple (1 apple)
¾oz (25g) of hazelnuts, chopped

Grate the apple or slice it thinly, sprinkle it with the chopped hazelnuts.

• EVENING MEAL

Garnished Pineapple Slices

10½oz (300g) of pineapple (½ pineapple)
5¼oz (150g) of mango
7oz (200g) of lychees

Peel the pineapple half saved from breakfast and remove the eyes. Cut the pineapple into thick slices (3 or 4). Use a sharp knife to remove carefully the hard cores from the pineapple slices, creating rings. Arrange the rings on a dish or plate. Peel the mango and cut it into long strips. Remove the peels and stones of the lychees. Garnish the pineapple rings with the mango strips and the lychees and add a mint or lemon balm leaf if so desired.

- BEFORE BEDTIME

1½–1¾oz (40–50g) of comb honey
herb tea

Day 4

Shopping List
1 pineapple
1 peach or apple
1 apricot or kiwi
¾oz (25g) of chopped hazelnuts
⅓oz (10g) of sunflower seeds
⅓oz (10g) of pumpkin seeds
⅓oz (10g) of brazil nuts
2 tomatoes
1 sprig of parsley
fresh herbs (basil, lovage)
7fl oz (200ml) of vegetable stock
1 small lettuce (you will only need ⅓oz or 10g)
1 spear of chicory
⅔oz (20g) of green celery (stalk, no leaves)
1 large avocado
½ lemon
5¼oz (150g) of cottage cheese (20 per cent fat)
1 orange
1 mandarin
1¾oz (50g) of grapes

- ON GETTING UP

1–2tbsp (15–30ml) of pollen

• BREAKFAST

Summery Pineapple Salad

10½oz (300g) of pineapple
5¼oz (150g) of peach or 5¼oz (150g) of apple (1 peach or 1 apple)
1¾oz (50g) of apricot or 3oz (80g) of kiwi (1 apricot or 1 kiwi)
⅓oz (10g) of wheat germ

Cut the pineapple in half (breadthwise) and save one half for the evening meal. Peel the other half, remove the eyes and the hard core and cut the flesh into small pieces. Rinse and/or peel the peach and the apricot and cut them into small pieces too. Mix all the fruits and sprinkle the whole with wheat germ.

• MID-MORNING

Nut–Seed Mix

⅓oz (10g) of sunflower seeds
⅓oz (10g) of pumpkin seeds
⅓oz (10g) of brazil nuts

Mix the sunflower seeds with the pumpkin seeds and the brazil nuts. Eat this mix with the fingers.

• MIDDAY MEAL

To start:

Fresh Tomato Soup

10½oz (300g) of tomato (2 tomatoes)
fresh parsley, basil and lovage, rinsed
7fl oz (200ml) of vegetable stock
optional herbs

Blanch the tomatoes in hot water, so that you can easily remove the skins. Cut the tomatoes into cubes and put them in the liquidizer (blender). Mix them together with rinsed fresh herbs. Add the hot stock and optional herbs.

Main course:

Chicory with a Spicy Avocado Sauce

a few leaves of lettuce
3½ (100g) of chicory
⅔oz (20g) of green celery (stalk)
5¼oz (150g) of avocado
1½ tsp (7.5ml) of mayonnaise
½ clove of garlic
a few drops of lemon juice
(optional: a pinch of curry powder)

Rinse and dry the lettuce and arrange it on a plate. Rinse the chicory and cut off the bottom of the spear so that the leaves come off. Arrange these leaves on the plate with the lettuce. Rinse the celery stalk and cut it into pieces. Peel the avocado and purée it together with the pieces of celery, the mayonnaise, the garlic, the lemon juice (and the curry powder). Pour this sauce over the chicory leaves in order to fill them.

• TEATIME

Cottage Cheese

5¼oz (150g) of cottage cheese (20 per cent fat)

Mix 1 tbsp (15ml) of wheat germ with a bowl of cottage cheese.

- EVENING MEAL

Citrus Cocktail

5¼oz (150g) of orange (1 orange)
3oz (80g) of mandarin (1 mandarin)
10½oz (300g) of pineapple (½ pineapple)
1¾oz (50g) of grapes
some fresh mint leaves
¾oz (25g) of whipped cream

Scoop out the pineapple half with a sharp knife and cut the flesh into pieces. Peel the orange in such a way that the flesh becomes visible; do this above a bowl, in order to catch the juice. Now segment the orange by cutting in between the visible membranes with a sharp knife. Peel the mandarin and separate its pieces. Mix them with the orange and pineapple pieces. Fill the pineapple half with this mixture and garnish it with whipped cream and mint leaves.

- BEFORE BEDTIME

1½oz (40–50g) of comb honey
herb tea

Day 5

Shopping List
1 melon
1 pineapple
⅔oz (20g) of mixed lettuce (small bag)
1 spear of chicory
⅔oz (20g) of garden cress
10½oz (300g) of tomato (2)
½ cucumber
1 red or yellow pepper

a few sprigs of chervil
7oz (200g) of yoghurt
1 pear
1 mandarin
⅔oz (20g) of almond flakes
wheatgerm (you will only need a pinch)

• ON GETTING UP

1–2tbsp (15–30ml) of pollen

• BREAKFAST

Honeydew Melon
24½oz (700g) of honeydew melon (1 melon)

Cut the honeydew melon in half, remove the seeds and scoop the
flesh out with a melon scoop. Put the melon balls in a bowl.
Remove the remaining flesh with a spoon, then fill the melon
halves with the melon balls. They may be sprinkled with some
fruit juice.

• MID-MORNING

Pineapple Juice
10½oz (300g) of pineapple (½ pineapple)

Use a liquidizer (blender) to squeeze the juice out of the half
pineapple, leaving the other half for the evening meal.

• MIDDAY MEAL

To start:

Fresh Vegetable Salad
⅔oz (20g) of mixed lettuce
3½oz (100g) of chicory

⅔oz (20g) of garden cress, rinsed
⅔oz (20g) of mayonnaise (1tbsp (15ml))
optional fresh herbs

Rinse and dry the lettuce, shred it and put it in a bowl. Clean the
chicory, shred it and add it to the lettuce. Mix the chicory with
the lettuce strips and add the mayonnaise. Garnish with the
rinsed garden cress and the fresh herbs.

Main course:

Southern Tomato Salad

10½oz (300g) of tomato (2 tomatoes)
7oz (200g) of cucumber (½ cucumber)
2½oz (70g) of red or yellow pepper (1 pepper)
a few sprigs of chervil, shredded
⅔oz (20ml) of vinaigrette (4 tsp safflower oil, 1 tsp of mustard,
    lemon juice)
⅙oz (5g) of garlic (1 clove)
herbs (basil, oregano, mixed herbs)

Rinse the tomatoes and cut them into slices or wedges. Peel the
cucumber, remove the seeds if necessary and slice it thinly. Rinse
the pepper, remove the seeds and cut it into cubes or strips. Mix
the vegetables in a bowl and sprinkle them with the shredded
chervil. Prepare a vinaigrette consisting of mustard, oil and lemon
juice to taste. Then add the crushed clove of garlic and the dried
or fresh herbs. Pour this dressing on the tomato salad and mix
everything well. Refrigerate the salad for 1–2 hours.

• TEATIME

Yoghurt

7oz (200g) of yoghurt

Stir a tablespoon of wheat germ into a dish of yoghurt.

- EVENING MEAL

Pineapple with Almond Flakes

10½oz (300g) of pineapple (½ pineapple)
5¼oz (150g) of pear (1 pear)
3oz (80g) of mandarin (1 mandarin)
⅔oz (20g) of almond flakes (2 tbsp (30ml))

Scoop out the pineapple half left from the mid-morning, remove
the hard core and cut the flesh into pieces. Add peeled pieces of
pear and mandarin to the pineapple flesh. Mix the fruit well and
fill the pineapple half with it. Garnish with almond flakes.

- BEFORE BEDTIME

1½–1¾oz (40–50g) of comb honey
herb tea

Day 6

Shopping List
1 pineapple
10½oz (300g) of mango
5½oz (160g) of kiwi
1¾oz (50g) of celery (stalk only)
3½oz (100g) of asparagus
1 spear of chicory
1 pepper
1¾oz (50g) of low-fat yoghurt (1.5 per cent)
1¾oz (50g) of mixed lettuce (1 small bag)
3½oz (100g) of mushrooms
⅙oz (5g) of garden cress (1 punnet)
1 avocado (you will only need to use ½)
1 orange
1½oz (40g) of cottage cheese (2tbsp (30ml))

5¼oz (150g) of gooseberries
5 lychees
¾oz (25g) of whipped cream

- ON GETTING UP

1–2tbsp (15–30ml) of pollen

- BREAKFAST

Tropical Fruit Dish

10½oz (300g) of pineapple (½ pineapple)
10½oz (300g) of mango
3oz (80g) of kiwi

Peel the half pineapple and remove the hard core and eyes. Cut the flesh into strips. Cut the mango lengthwise, right to the stone. Then use a sharp knife to carve the mango: make slanting scores in the flesh, without damaging the skin of the mango – don't cut through the skin! Then make some more scores at right angles to the other scores, still not cutting through the skin. Hold the mango in such a way that the skin is at the bottom and the flesh on top. Use your thumbs to push the skin upwards in order to turn the mango inside out. The mango has turned into a mango-hedgehog. Peel the kiwi and slice it. Arrange the pineapple strips, the mango-hedgehog and the kiwi slices on a dish.

- MID-MORNING

Pineapple Juice

10½oz (300g) of pineapple (½ pineapple)

Use a liquidizer (blender) to squeeze the juice out of the pineapple.

• MIDDAY MEAL

To start:

Vegetable Dip

1¾oz (50g) celery (stalk only)
3½oz (100g) of asparagus, raw or blanched
3½oz (100g) of chicory
2½oz (70g) of pepper (1 pepper)
yoghurt dip (1¾oz (50g) of yoghurt mixed with fresh and/or dried herbs)

Clean the vegetables. Cut the celery stalk into pieces of about 2in (5cm). Leave the asparagus whole, separate the chicory leaves and cut the pepper into strips. Arrange the vegetables on a dish and serve together with the yoghurt dip.

Main course:

Mushroom Salad

1¾oz (50g) of mixed lettuces
3½oz (100g) of mushrooms
⅙oz (5g) of garden cress
2¾oz (75g) of avocado (½ avocado)
2 tbsp (30ml) of mayonnaise
parsley

Rinse and dry the lettuce and arrange it on a plate. Clean the mushrooms and slice them. Arrange the slices on the lettuce, garnish with garden cress and serve it with an avocado dip. For the dip, mash the avocado with the mayonnaise and add a squeeze of lemon juice and chopped parsley.

- TEATIME

Stuffed Orange

2¾oz (75g) of orange (about ½ orange)
1½oz (40g) of cottage cheese
A pinch of wheatgerm

Scoop out the orange half and cut the flesh into pieces. Mix those with the cottage cheese and the wheat germ, and stuff the orange with this mixture.

- EVENING MEAL

Fruit Salad

5¼oz (150g) of gooseberries
3oz (80g) of kiwi
5¼oz (150g) of lychees (5 lychees)
Juice of ½ sweet orange
¾oz (25g) of whipped cream

Rinse the gooseberries. Peel the kiwi and cut it into pieces. Peel the lychees and remove their stones. Mix the fruit well and add the orange juice to it. Serve with whipped cream.

- BEFORE BEDTIME

1½–1¾oz (40–50g) of comb honey
herb tea

Day 7

Shopping List
1 pineapple
16oz (450g) of cherries or 1 pear
5¼oz (150g) of apples (1 apple)

1¾oz (50g) of whipped cream
5¼oz (150g) of cottage cheese (20 per cent fat)
1 cucumber
1¾oz (50g) of yoghurt
¾oz (25g) of sour cream (1 tbsp (15ml))
⅔oz (20g) of safflower oil
5¼oz (150g) of tomatoes
7fl oz (200ml) of vegetable stock
14oz (400g) of summer fruit (bilberries, raspberries, strawberries, lychees)
or 14oz (400g) of winter fruit (apples, pears, oranges, mandarins)

- ON GETTING UP

1–2 tbsp (15–30ml) of pollen

- BREAKFAST

Cherry/Apple Pineapple

10½oz (300g) of pineapple (½ pineapple)
5¼oz (150g) of cherries (or 1 pear)
5¼oz (150g) of apple (1 apple) or 1 mandarin
¾oz (25g) of whipped cream

Cut the pineapple in half, lengthwise. Scoop it out, remove the hard core and cut the flesh into pieces. Rinse and stone the cherries and add them to the pineapple. Peel and core the apple and cut it into small pieces. Add the apple to the pineapple–cherry combination. Fill the pineapple half with this mixture.

- MID-MORNING

Cottage Cheese

5¼oz (150g) of cottage cheese (20 per cent fat)

Mix 1tbsp (15ml) of wheat germ with a bowl of cottage cheese.

- MIDDAY MEAL

To start:

Tomato–Cucumber Soup

5¼oz (150g) of tomatoes (peeled)
7oz (200g) of cucumber (peeled)
herbs (basil, mixed herbs, oregano)
7fl oz (200ml) of vegetable stock

Put the peeled tomatoes and cucumber in the liquidizer (blender). Add the chopped fresh or dried herbs. Finally, add 7fl oz (200ml) of hot stock and serve the soup hot.

Main course:

Tzatziki

7oz (200g) of cucumber
1¾oz (50g) of yoghurt
⅔oz (20g) of sour cream
1 or ½ clove of garlic
a few drops of lemon juice
4 tsp (20ml) of safflower oil

Purée the peeled and deseeded cucumber, put it in a colander and leave it there for about 20 minutes. Mix the other ingredients and add the puréed cucumber to this mixture. Refrigerate for six hours. Serve it with a salad of tomato, lettuce, watercress, etc.

- TEATIME

Pineapple Juice

10½oz (300g) of pineapple (½ pineapple)

Use a liquidizer (blender) to squeeze the juice out of the pineapple.

- EVENING MEAL

Summer Fruit Salad

14oz (400g) of summer fruit (bilberries, raspberries, strawberries, lychees)
or 14oz (400g) of winter fruit (apples, pears, oranges, mandarins)
¾oz (25g) of whipped cream

Rinse or peel the fruits (cut up the large pieces) and mix them. Add some whipped cream if desired.

- BEFORE BEDTIME

1½–1¾oz (40–50g) of comb honey
herb tea

Dressings

Yoghurt Dressing

Mix 1¾oz (50g) of yoghurt with 1tsp (5ml) of safflower oil and add optional fresh or dried herbs (basil, oregano, parsley, chives, thyme, garlic, mixed herbs, etc.).

Yoghurt–Mayonnaise Dressing

Mix 2 parts of mayonnaise with 1 part of yoghurt and add optional fresh or fried herbs.

Vinaigrette

Take 4 tsp (20ml) of safflower oil and add a little bit of mustard. Add wine vinegar or lemon juice until the vinaigrette has the right sourness, according to your own taste. Add optional fresh or dried herbs.

Oil Dressing

Take 4 tsp (20ml) of safflower oil and add fresh herbs (such as dill, thyme, basil, lovage, etc.) to it. If fresh herbs are not available, replace them with dried herbs. Let the herb–oil mixture steep at least overnight and remove the herbs before using it.

Herb Tea

The following are recipes for two mixed herb teas that are very suitable for supporting the diet.

A general-purpose diet-supporting blend

1oz (30g) of lavender blossom
⅔oz (25g) of aniseed
½oz (15g) of (stinging-)nettle
½oz (15g) of horsetail
½oz (15g) of camomile blossom
3½oz (100g) total weight

Have this herb mixture prepared by a herbalist. These herbs can be bought separately and mixed in the proportions given.

Use 1tsp (5ml) of this mixture for each cup of tea. Pour boiling water on it and let it brew for 10 minutes, then strain and sweeten with honey to taste. Drink 2–5 cups a day.

Purifying Tea for Chemotherapy

Patients who have been treated with cytostatics are usually advised to drink large quantities of water. The water allows the kidneys to get rid of the chemical substances as quickly as possible. There is also a lot of cell waste that has to be removed. A herb tea works much better than water because the herbs activate the kidneys and the bladder and drain the liquid from the tissues. Here is a good herb recipe:

¾oz (25g) of horsetail
¾oz (25g) of birch leaf
¾oz (25g) of (stinging-)nettle
¾oz (25g) of elderberry blossom
3oz (100g) total weight (Equivalent in ounces per 100g varies slightly because of approximations for small amounts.)

How to prepare the tea is described in the previous recipe.

After every chemotherapy treatment, drink 1 or 1.5 litres of this tea, for 3–5 days. It is also recommended that pineapple juice be taken after a chemotherapy treatment, or that a monodiet consisting of pineapple be followed. Increased use of pollen to 1½oz (40g) or 2oz (60g) a day for the 3–5 days that precede the treatment should also be included in this diet.

Month:	J	F	M	A	M	J	J	A	S	O	N	D
Apricot						■	■	■				
Pineapple	□	□	□						■	■	■	■
Apple	■	■	■	■	■		■	■	■	■	■	■
Banana	■	■	■	■	■	■	■	■	■	■	■	■
Bilberry					□	■	■	□				
Cactus fruit	□	□	□	□						□	□	□
Lemon	■	■	■	■	■	■						
Grape	□	□			□			■	■	■	□	□
Feijoa			□	□					□			
Raspberry							■	■	□			
Grapefruit	■	■	■	■	■	■	■	■	■	■	■	■
Honeydew melon	□	□	□	□				■	■	□	□	□
Persimmon			□	□				□	□	□	□	
Cherry						■	■	□				
Kiwi	■	■	■		■	■	■	■	■	■	■	■
Lychee	□	□	□	□	□							□
Mandarin	■	■	□							□	■	■
Mango	■	■	■	■	■	■	■	■	■	■	■	■
Melon	□	□	□	□	□	□	□	□	□	□	□	□
Papaya	□	□	□	□	□	□	□	□	□	□	□	□
Passion fruit	□	□	□	□	□	□	□	□	□	□	□	□
Pear		□						■	■	■		
Peach	□	□	□	□	□	■	■	■	■			
Plum	□	□	□	□	□		■	■	■			
Redcurrant						□	■	■				
Raisins	□	□								■	■	■
Orange	■	■	■	■	■		□			□		■
Gooseberry					□	■	■					
Blackcurrant							■	■				

■ Months with a high supply   □ Months with a low supply

Figure 11 *Chart indicating the seasonal availability of different fruits*

Chapter 7

Never Lose Hope

Faith and Hope

When cancer strikes, the patient finds him- or herself in dire straits, in a situation ruled by fear, insecurity and – most of all – despair. The Dries diet can convert that despair into hope. Whoever follows the diet as it is described here, will get better in no time at all. And it is exactly that improvement that stimulates the hope. In most cases, we can already see that the diet is working after only four weeks. A blood analysis or an examination by a specialist will confirm that. Such a good start incites the patients sufficiently to continue following the diet and to apply it even better. They get used to the diet. They know where to find the ingredients and how to assess their quality. They start to really like the diet and do not miss their old eating habits any more. Their acquaintances start to notice that they look better, are able to do more and are happier, because they know they are on the right track. Full of enthusiasm, the patients look forward to the next examination. Like mountaineers, they climb the steep mountainside and go for the top.

The watchword is: carry on, grit the teeth and look forward! The diet not only provides sublimed solar power (bio-energy), but also psychological power. That is because the body is purified and functions better, and especially because of the increase in bio-energy. After all, body and mind are one. Every physical improvement results in more psychological energy. The Dries diet has both physical and psychological effects. Not only the dieters notice that, but also those around them, and that is the best stimulus.

This enthusiasm contrasts sharply with the cheerless mood and the negative attitude of many oncologists, surgeons or other medical specialists. They are extremely careful with their statements regarding improvements. That is understandable: every day they see how difficult it is to treat cancer and how unreliable the prognosis can be. Temporary improvements may just as well turn into a deterioration of the condition in no time. When they are suddenly confronted with such good and lasting results, they do not understand what is happening. Even if the patients tell them they are following the Dries diet, they still cannot believe that this use of food is capable of producing such results. Some are speechless, others say that there is no proof and still others are indifferent. One physician was extremely surprised when he found that the tumour (that had been the size of a hen's egg) in An Daems, one of his patients, had disappeared. When An's husband told him that An was following the Dries diet, the physician said: 'It's always wise to have two strings to one's bow.' After that he avoided every conversation about food. Seven years later, An Daems started to suffer from epileptic fits. The physician immediately told her it was the tumour again. The neurologist in hospital shared his opinion, but the examination indicated that the scar of the tumour had barely grown in those seven years. One millimetre at the most is what they diagnosed.

When speaking of An Daems, by the way, we are discussing a real person with a real problem being treated; in this chapter and earlier, other real people's problems are also discussed. In order to protect their privacy, as is often done, we have used pseudonyms which we hope will not create embarrassment for anyone coincidentally by the same name.

Such positive results as in An's case are often considered spontaneous recoveries. Spontaneous recoveries are not unknown in the medical world. It has happened in the past that someone was doomed to die and still recovered. There is no explanation for that. Nevertheless there are three important factors that can play a part in spontaneous recoveries: the self-healing mechanism, the power of the mind and the survival instinct. Everyone possesses a self-healing power, a mechanism that will do anything to cure an illness. This means the body is capable of healing itself. The strong longing to survive, to be healthy again, can influence the self-healing mechanism. The survival instinct is a force that is underestimated far too often. Because the Dries diet operates so close to the natural needs of human beings, we may assume that it influences the survival instinct and that it strengthens our natural powers. Just like the diet, positive thoughts also stimulate the self-healing mechanism. The self-healing mechanism is closely related to instinct in general. From naturopathy, it is easy to explain a spontaneous recovery. Just look at animals that roam freely in their natural habitats every day.

Good advice

There are undoubtedly people in the dieter's direct surroundings who care about him or her and who give him or her good advice. They say that they have read somewhere that certain foodstuffs or herbs are very good. Sometimes they are talking from their own experience and sometimes they know someone who has been able to benefit from that advice. But the dieter must be wary of such well-meant suggestions, and should keep to the diet and not deviate from it. The Dries diet is based on bio-energetic science and I doubt that these would-be advisers are familiar with that science. Foodstuffs that are not part of the seven groups are not necessarily bad. They just do not have enough influence on the dieter's illness, or we would of course have included them in our recommendations.

The advice from other people is often very negative. Comments such as: 'You should be careful!', 'What do you think you are doing?', 'It's irresponsible.' and 'Do you have any scientific proof?' are very common. Patients who have only just started the diet and who cannot expect immediate improvement yet, often meet with great opposition on the part of relatives or other family members, especially during the first period. Many people are worried about the patients when they start to lose weight, which happens mainly during those first weeks. That is very unfortunate, because it is exactly during that period that cancer patients need the most encouragement. On the other hand I can understand why people react in that way; they are worried, and react out of sheer ignorance. The best weapon against these negative opinions is objective information. Those other people should be advised to read this book or one of my other health books. It will give them new insight.

As soon as the patients are clearly improving, all those negative comments disappear. By that time, people understand what the power of the Dries diet is. They are not as critical of the difference between this diet and traditional food any more. They understand how the whole food industry can be an enormous threat to the health of mankind.

There are also families that adapt to the situation very well. I can name many wonderful examples of relatives who support cancer patients in every possible way. Sometimes the whole family switches over to the Dries diet, and everyone starts the day with a fruit breakfast or eats a fruit meal during the day. In one family I know, the mother shares lunch with her ailing son Joop, and in the evening Joop's father shares dinner with him. The involvement of relatives is very important: they also have to respect the nutritional rules and the natural way of life. It is the change of mentality that has a stimulating influence on the recovery process.

Duration of the Diet

Generally, everyone follows the diet for three months. After that the diet is continued, adapted or made more flexible, depending on the improvement of the condition. A diet as strict as this one need not be followed for the rest of the dieter's life. As soon as the medical examination has proven the disease is under control, the dieter can gradually switch to ordinary healthy food again. It is obvious that a former cancer patient has to eat healthy food for the rest of his or her life, but does that not apply to everyone? Many people watch their food, have large amounts of fruit every day and eat neither meat nor fish. They use recipes like the ones you can find in *200 New Food Combining Recipes* by Inge Dries (also published by Element), a book which contains tasty recipes that help to apply the rules of food combining spontaneously. Why would a cancer patient who has been lucky enough to recover from his or her illness not do the same? Healthy food is the best way to prevent cancer or a relapse.

At parties or on holiday

Sometimes people who are following the diet are invited to a party or dinner. It usually makes them feel very uncomfortable, because the food at those parties is likely to be not as healthful as their diet demands. On the other hand, they do not want to refuse the invitation, because a party is always a very special occasion. Just setting aside the diet and participating is not a good solution. The dieter cannot just go to a party and destroy what he or she has worked so hard for. The dieter cannot just start polluting the body – that has become so clean by now – by reducing the amount of bio-energy that has been built up with so much determination. Such risks must be avoided. Most dieters understand that, but they still want a good solution. The people who have sent the invitation can be informed of the dieter's problem: they can be told that he or she is following a strict diet from which no deviation is permitted. An acceptable party-time meal can be suggested to the host or hostess: a tasty starter, a side-dish, a soup, a main course and a dessert. Whoever is doing the cooking will understand and may even be happy to prepare something exceptional for one of the guests. The dieting party-goer should ask to be served first though, or at least at the same time as the others, in order to not have to wait till the very last with an empty plate. That is very embarrassing because by then everyone will have noticed. They will possibly ask awkward questions. As can be seen, however, the dieter can participate fully in the party.

When the dieter is travelling or on a holiday, the same problems can arise. A relaxed holiday is a good therapy in itself. The best thing is a self-catering holiday home where the dieter can prepare his or her own food. A restaurant likely cannot be expected to provide daily suitable dietary foodstuffs such as we recommend. In Mediterranean countries and the southern hemisphere there is an abundance of fresh, ripe fruit during the summer. It's even advisable, perhaps, to go to somewhere with a southern climate during the summer. But busy tourist areas are to be avoided in favour of quiet surroundings: for example, mountain areas where the air is clean and where it is less hot. A clean, natural environment has a favourable influence on the recovery process. The dieter must try to relax during the holiday, and to enjoy the beautiful moments as much as possible. I have met patients who showed remarkable improvement after three or four weeks of holiday. On the other had, there were also patients who returned worn out and exhausted from a quite tumultuous holiday. The scorching sun and the concrete megaprojects for mass tourism are not sensible holiday destinations for people dealing with ill health, who should try to find peace and quiet and to feel a connection with nature, because if they succeed in doing that, they can at least find strength to recover.

All over the world there are wonderful places where peace and quiet can be found, in which recuperation can be encouraged. One ideal holiday destination for European cancer patients could be Madeira. On this Portuguese island far away in the Atlantic Ocean it never gets hotter than 30°C, but it never gets colder than 18°C either. (These days, of course, holidaymakers will keep in mind the sensible rules about covering up against the sun's effects on their bodies.) Madeira is an eternally green island with a wide variety of different fruits. At the market of Funchal, there are many fruit merchants from whom to buy the fruit needed. There are not many tourists on Madeira and one hopes that it will always be that way. The air is reasonably clean there and there seems to be hardly any heavy industry on the island, but there are beautiful places to relax or to go for a walk. Cancer patients who are very mobile, who need no medical attention and who do not belong to a high-risk group should by all means go for a holiday. They do not even have to go far. It is good just to be in a different environment away from home, away from all worries. But such patients must make sure to not exhaust themselves. The recovery process demands a lot of energy and that is why care must be taken over what is done with that energy. Intense physical exertion is to be avoided, as are long hikes in the mountains or rambling, excursions or tiring sports and long, exhausting visits to museums or other monuments. Daily exercise, untaxing sports and just being busy are good as long as these activities do not demand too much effort.

I have personally witnessed something quite remarkable: one of my patients, who is suffering from Kahler's disease (bone cancer), is in perfect condition thanks to the Dries cancer diet combined with the beneficial effects of trips away. He went on holiday three times and after every holiday the number of white blood cells in his blood had increased dramatically. There exists no form of medication that can increase the number of blood cells after chemotherapy so the only explanation for the increase must be the holidays themselves. As soon as he got back home the number of white blood cells dropped again. This shows how important a holiday can be for someone suffering from cancer.

This holiday time is good for people to discover silence, learn how to enjoy it and take courage from it. A lot of people are afraid of silence. They fear it will make them have negative thoughts, but that is not true. Once silence is discovered, so also will be the healing power in oneself and, also, a way to enjoy life.

Food at work

When I was explaining the cancer diet to a patient named Piet Jansen, he made the following comment: 'It must be difficult to take that kind of food to work.' I was speechless with amazement when I heard this, because Piet's wife had told me that he had no chance of recovery. Piet had a serious form of lung cancer and he refused to undergo treatment. I advised him to take sick leave and to start living in another way. Piet visited me very often and he was very pleased about his new way of life. In spite of his serious illness, he still lived for quite a long period of time. When Piet was finally hospitalized, they were surprised he had managed to live that long in such good condition. The medical care they gave him went by very smoothly. For Piet, it had been a good choice to refuse the heavy chemotherapy. Unfortunately, nobody knows beforehand how his or her illness will develop.

There are patients who want to go back to work as quickly as possible. Sometimes they work part-time. They are afraid they will get bored or lose contact with their colleagues if they do not go to work. And sometimes they just want to forget about their illness as soon as possible. When someone becomes ill with cancer, he or she often has many visitors during the first weeks, but because cancer is a long-lasting disease, the frequency of those visits drops rapidly. The patient feels abandoned and lonely. Nevertheless every cancer patient needs to rest and relax as much as possible. I have known several terminal patients who kept on working up to a few weeks before their deaths. Some just worked to be busy, but others took refuge in their work. They pretended nothing was wrong, and that is seldom a good solution.

When the patient goes to work, it is also important for him or her not to overexert: no extra efforts, no great responsibility and certainly not too much worry. Men often have the tendency to continue their professional life as before, but they forget that it costs them a lot of energy, even though they do not notice that immediately. But it is equally wrong to sit in a chair and slowly waste away the entire day. I have also seen cancer patients whose lives suddenly changed completely. They adopted a totally different way of life. They spent their time in a useful and sensible way. If there is a desire to go to work, there is a need to adapt the diet. Without deviating from the diet, all the necessary ingredients must be included in it. Fruit in its natural form can be eaten anywhere. Vegetable salad can be brought to work in small containers, as long as it can be refrigerated. Processed food must never be taken to work, though, because of the risk of fermentation. Nuts, almonds, pollen and herb tea at work can be used without causing too much trouble for others.

Who Will Benefit from the Dries Diet?

The Dries diet is suitable for all cancer patients. It does not matter what kind of cancer they have. There are many kinds of cancer and they all have specific properties, but as a disease cancer is always the same. The kind of cancer depends on the way in which the cancer manifests itself. The Dries diet does not affect the specific kind of cancer, but its nature. The Dries diet stimulates the self-healing mechanism by increasing the human bio-energy and the electric potential of the cells, which leads to a depolarization of the cancer cells. People have to see the recovery process from a point of view that is different from the one they are used to. The Dries diet increases bio-energy by purifying the organism on the one hand and by making the patient use foodstuffs with a high bio-energetic value on the other hand.

The affected organ – that is, the organ in which the tumour has manifested itself – is not necessarily a weak or sick organ. That is why it is not always necessary to give extra support to that organ. Nevertheless it may be useful to add foodstuffs that have a favourable influence on that organ to the diet. We do want to mention that the Dries diet has a general effect, though. We only adapt the diet individually and after a personal discussion with the patient involved.

The Dries diet can be applied at all times, even when the disease is already under control after chemotherapy or a number of radiation treatments. Surgery, chemotherapy and radiotherapy have a destructive influence on the defence mechanism. That is why it is always advisable to apply the Dries diet very strictly for at least three months.

By applying the Dries diet, a patient can defend against a possible relapse, although unfortunately nothing can give absolute certainty. But if the diet is applied, the chance of the cancer recurring is reduced considerably; and if it does happen anyway, the dieter has more chance of recovery.

If the cancer has already spread, it is also a good idea to start applying the Dries diet. Even though the prognosis may be hopeless, there is always a chance of sudden change and that is an opportunity the patient cannot afford to miss. Cancer is an unpredictable disease and that can also be interpreted in a positive sense: three years after a mastectomy, a cancer patient named Marieke (whose surname I blush to say I do not remember) was told she had metastasis in lungs and liver. In spite of negative comments, she decided to start following the Dries diet on the advice of her physician. Marieke recovered completely.

It is also possible that the side-effects of the regular treatment are so serious that the Dries diet cannot repair the damage, in spite of its positive effects. Even in those cases, it is advisable to start following the diet. The disease will take a completely different course. I once met a cancer patient, Julia Thijs, whom everyone had already given up on, whose condition was extremely serious. Julia was sitting in front of me in her wheelchair, and it was my opinion that comforting words would do her more good than my diet. Nevertheless, she decided to follow the diet. Five weeks later Julia was in my waiting room again, but this time without a wheelchair. I did not recognize her at first, she had changed so much. Her husband showed me Julia's medical records, which stated that there had been significant changes. Especially the statistics of the blood analyses showed remarkable improvements. Julia's physician had drawn up a chart in order to scale down the amount of painkillers she was taking. After all, the painkillers had become redundant. Unfortunately Julia's system had already been weakened to such an extent that she was not able to recover any more, and she died a few months later. The months during which Julia had been applying the Dries diet had been the most bearable months of her illness. Like her, other terminal patients who have enough strength left, and who still have a reasonable appetite, can still benefit from following the diet, even if recovery is not one of the possibilities. The diet can lengthen their lives and – more importantly – improve the quality of their lives. They do not need medical treatments or heavy drugs any more, or at least not to the same extent.

Patients with a stomach carcinoma, whose stomachs have been removed either completely or partially, can apply the Dries diet without any problems, provided that they adapt the diet a little. The best thing for them to do is to eat very small amounts very often. They will soon notice that the diet causes fewer problems for them than ordinary food. Stoma patients can switch over to the diet without any problems. Generally they claim this diet causes a lot fewer problems for them than industrial food does. They do have to be careful about using overripe fruit, though. Overripe fruit easily ferments. The best thing for them to do is to sprinkle the fruit with a lot of lemon juice. This will reduce the fermentation. Combining sour with sweet fruit is also advisable in order to reach the same objective.

The Dries diet can also be used as a means by which to prevent cancer. In that case it is enough to follow the diet for two or three weeks, but it should be repeated annually, preferably during summer when there is an abundance of fruit.

Who will not benefit from the Dries diet?

The Dries diet is not suitable for cancer patients who are diabetic at the same time, even though such a condition is not common.

It happens that these cancer patients cannot use the diet because of the large amounts of fruit and honey of which it consists. Their blood absorbs the simple sugars much too quickly, which makes their dextrose level rise. If they request it, and after a personal conversation, we are always willing to compose an adapted diet for diabetic patients. The same goes for patients who have had operations on the pancreas: the part that is responsible for the production of insulin may have been removed, which means they too are diabetic.

The diet is not suitable for patients who are not allowed to use sugar, or are allowed only limited amounts of sugar, for whatever reason. And, as has been said before, it is not suitable for people who are suffering from anorexia or malnutrition either. These people need a strengthening diet in order to normalize their body weight. Only after having achieved a weight normalization can they apply the Dries diet. Kidney patients whose kidney capacity is low and who are supposed to stick to a low-potassium diet should refrain from applying the Dries diet. A kidney carcinoma, however, is not always a reason not to apply the diet – if the kidney carcinoma does not interfere with the kidney function, which sometimes is the case, the diet is in fact very beneficial. When in doubt, the patient can consult a kidney specialist. If there are allergies to certain kinds of food, those kinds of food can be excluded from the diet. Finally, the Dries diet is not suitable for people who are not open to its philosophy: nutritional therapy requires the full cooperation of the patient.

If there are any problems during application of the diet, a GP should be consulted.

Additional Pain Relief and Possible Therapies

Fighting the pain

Even though cancer in itself does not cause any pain, any of many complications can cause serious pains. Cancer patients who are following the Dries diet sometimes ask me if they are allowed to use painkillers. They fear painkillers will harm the effects of the diet. Even though chemical drugs always lead to pollution of the metabolism, the use of them cannot always be avoided. Suffering pain is not only annoying but it also uses up a lot of energy. People who are in a lot of pain tend to lose weight easily. Very often the use of painkillers is a necessity. It should be recalled, however, that the diet gets rid of the toxic substances quite quickly. That purifying effect can be intensified by use of a purifying tea, as when the patient is undergoing chemotherapy, and can be done for all the chemical medication prescribed. The better the diet works, the lesser the need for chemical medication. If it is desired to reduce the use of medication, a GP should be consulted first.

Relaxation therapy

It has often been said that cancer is a very emotional disease. That undoubtedly has to do with its life-threatening nature. The fact that no one is prepared for it can create an atmosphere of panic and stress. The uncertainty and the powerless attitude of the people who surround the patient, because nobody has a solution, only worsen the entire situation. Within a very short period of time, several very important decisions have to be made. The changes within the family, the diet itself, etc. are all factors that will cause stress. Cancer is regularly accompanied by sorrow, despair and disappointment. Luckily for many people, they have the shoulder of their partner or a friend to cry on.

Stress and other emotional disorders use up much energy. That is why it is important for cancer patients to control their emotions and to avoid stress. Even healthy people are almost literally drained emotionally during a stress situation, so it can only be surmised what happens to cancer patients. All of this is understandable with the knowledge that stress proclaims a state of emergency and triggers defence mechanisms. Stress warns against all kinds of dangers or possible dangers. Not only the disease itself is a danger, but also everything that goes with it. If suffering from stress, the patient has an increased energy consumption – that is, an abnormally high consumption of sugars, vitamins and minerals. Too much stress undermines the favourable effects of the diet, as proven by extensive research. People who are capable of relaxing completely recover much sooner – not only from cancer but also from other diseases, even infectious diseases. If a patient is able to relax deeply, his or her bio-energy will increase and there will be a wealth of energy. That is why relaxation therapy is an important support, in addition to nutritional therapy. For that same reason a holiday, an excursion, some exercise or a relaxing sport are very useful, as mentioned earlier in this chapter.

Relaxing in a stressful situation is not that easy: it cannot be done on one's own. That is why relaxing should be done under the supervision of an experienced relaxation therapist.

Since I am a food therapist, many people who consult me have digestive problems. They ask me to tell them which diet is best for them. I often have to tell them that they do not have a digestive problem, but a stress problem; and that it is not food but relaxation that can cure their digestive system.

Of course good food is always indispensable; that is why I have been studying food for more than twenty years now. But at the same time I have also studied relaxation and have found that both therapies complement each other quite well. People often say that emotional disorders are the cause of cancer. Earlier in this book, I mentioned that no one can prove that. Nevertheless nearly everyone is convinced that emotional circumstances can easily cause cancer or cause it to break out more rapidly. The loss of a partner, a divorce, bankruptcy, the loss of a job, serious humiliations, etc. often preceed the onset of cancer. Often, cancer patients have introvert characters, bottling everything up and finding it difficult to express themselves. Sometimes they seem very extrovert but on the inside are very reserved, and camouflaged their characters by means of apparent openness: of them it could be said that people who open the gates of their front yards for everyone often keep their front doors locked.

Feelings are closely related to energy. Relaxation therapy is aimed at raising energy blockades, an important part of the recovery process. But increasing the bio-energy by means of food makes it a lot easier to achieve relaxation.

I have been working as a relaxation therapist for more than twenty years now and I have counselled thousands of patients, both individually and in groups, with biorelaxation, a very natural way to relax, even for cancer patients. Cancer patients do not need adapted exercises, because all the exercises have a favourable influence on their recovery process. Of course we can slightly adapt the biorelaxation exercises in such a way that they are more specifically tuned in to the patient's clinical picture or more specifically aimed at rescuing the patient from his or her illness. Regardless, the relaxation has to be very intense and the patients need to have a thorough mastery of the principles of biorelaxation. Those principles are: good respiration, adapted muscle relaxation, absence of thought (thinking of nothing), fixation, evoking subjective perceptions, imaginative extension, and autosuggestion or suggestion. Patients who have undergone surgery cannot do all these exercises, but that is not really a problem. There are enough exercises at their disposal.

Imaginative extension (or visualization) is especially important for cancer patients. Biorelaxation helps them to think more positively. Visualization and autosuggestion develop the power of the mind. In effect, the patients learn how to raise blockades so that an optimal flow of energy is created, very important for the recovery process. Relaxation therapy influences the sympathetic and the parasympathetic nervous systems. Stress disrupts the balance between the two systems, resulting in serious functional disorders. The entire human physiology is controlled by the sympathetic and the parasympathetic systems. When the function of the nervous systems is disrupted by stress or emotional disorders, one of these two will start to dominate. Digestion, metabolism, immunity, relaxation and rest are all

LCH = left cerebral hemisphere
RCH = right cerebral hemisphere
BS = brainstem

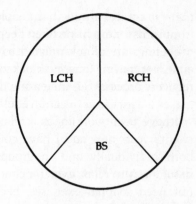

Figure 12 *Diagram of the brain: brain (L CH/R CH and Brainstem)*

controlled by the two systems. By relaxing deeply, the subject can not only save energy, but also create more energy because he or she has a better physiology.

Furthermore, I would like to point out that deep relaxation improves the interaction between the grey matter of the brain (cortex) and the brainstem. That is very important, since an overburdened cortex obstructs the brainstem, which is responsible for the five basic vital functions: eating, breathing, sleeping, sexuality and rest. A well-functioning brainstem stimulates the survival instinct, which means that it also stimulates the self-healing mechanism.

Finally, I would like to mention the interaction between the right and the left cerebral hemispheres. In Western societies, rational persons use the left cerebral hemisphere too much and emotional individuals – who often lack a sense of reality – are stuck in the right hemisphere. Biorelaxation therapy teaches how to use both hemispheres together, and that also influences the recovery process. I cannot emphasize enough how favourable the influence of adapted biorelaxation therapy on cancer patients can be. (My book *Biorelaxation* and the exercise cassettes can be ordered from my Dutch publisher, Arinus. For more information on stress and relaxation therapy, I recommend my *Stress Control,* also obtainable through the publisher.) In the United States, O Carl Simonton has broken new ground on this subject; various other researchers have proven that relaxation has a positive influence on recovery from cancer. I want especially to point out that relaxation therapy also has a favourable influence on the results of the diet, apart from its general influence. That is why relaxation therapy has a double effect.

Other Possible Therapies

Even though experience has taught me that food and biorelaxation are the two most important complementary therapies, there are many other possible alternative treatments. I want to mention those possibilities here because it may be useful to apply one or more of them. I sometimes meet cancer patients who are following a wide variety of alternative therapies, which does not necessarily mean they obtain better results. Over-consumption is completely wrong: it overburdens the body's extremely vulnerable mechanisms, which can no longer cope with any of the therapies. A patient has to be able to deal with his or her therapy or therapies. A therapy is an impulse and if you give too many impulses to an organism, it becomes over-stimulated. In Germany, it has been discovered that an excessive dose of immunizing medication weakens the defence mechanism instead of strengthening it. Unfortunately, overconsumption occurs quite often in the domain of alternative treatment. This is caused by quantitative thinking. The slogan 'More is better' is very established, very deep-rooted, also with respect to cancer patients. In naturopathy, it is not the quantity that is important, but the result of every impulse. Filling the stove with coal is not always enough: sometimes you have to use the poker to stir up the fire.

Colonic irrigation

This method involves rinsing the large intestine with lukewarm, clean water under a certain pressure. It is not a painful or annoying method; on the contrary, patients find that it gives a pleasant feeling of purity afterwards. The lavages take place while a special intestinal message is applied. Usually a number of lavages are spread over several weeks. This method completely cleans the intestinal wall and improves the digestion, which makes the diet work more efficiently. A clean intestine relieves the job of the liver: It is, after all, the liver that has to detoxify poisonous substances that are formed in the intestine. High lavages are to be greatly recommended, especially for cancer patients.

Fasting and juice (sap) cures

Fasting means completely abstaining from food for one to three weeks, during which time only spring water and herb tea may be taken. Fasting can sometimes be an efficient therapy in the fight against cancer, provided that the patient is not too emaciated or exhausted; fasting has to be done under supervision. A less severe method is the juice cure, in which liquid food is taken in the form of freshly squeezed juice. A juice cure does not have the same effect as fasting. While you are following the Dries diet, you can introduce one or more juice days by way of a change.

Homoeopathy

Homoeopathy is a frequently applied therapy that can support recovery from cancer. Experience has taught us that patients who combine the Dries cancer diet with homoeopathy can obtain striking results.

Anthroposophic medicine

Icador is a preparation made of mistletoe. It is used to support the recovery from cancer. Even though it is a much sought-after remedy, it is not likely to have a powerful effect. It is only a complementary remedy.

Biological preparations

In recent decades, scientists have developed dozens of preparations based on natural ingredients. The manufacturers admit that these preparations cannot cure cancer. The purpose of biological preparations is to strengthen or repair the defence mechanism – damaged by surgery, radiotherapy or chemotherapy – as much as possible.

A welcome note is that in the last few years we have made much progress, and the pharmaceuticals industry is now able to offer some very powerful preparations that play an important part in the biological fight against cancer.

Enzyme therapy

In Germany enzyme therapy has been used in the fight against cancer for years now. Enzymes are the weapons of the defence mechanism, making the blood more liquid and preventing metastasis. A good cancer therapy without enzymes is unthinkable, according to Dr R De Greef, a noted naturopath and food therapist in Belgium.[1]

[1] See Dr R De Greef, *Immunologie*, Arinus, Genk, 1992, *passim*.

Thymus extract

This extract consists of liquids derived from the thymus glands of calves specially bred for this purpose. Thymus extract is used to prevent illnesses, treat geriatric complaints, and generally support the defence mechanism. In this case thymus extract is used in the biological fight against cancer, but is not a specific cancer preparation. The same can be said about cell therapy.

Ozone therapy

This therapy involves taking a certain amount of blood from the patient, enriching it with ozone and then injecting it back into the bloodstream, where the ozone is converted into oxygen. Ozone therapy is said to trigger a chain reaction of free radicals which kills weakened cells, viruses and bacteria. Before applying this therapy, one has to make sure that the healthy cells in the body are strong enough to resist free radicals. That check on healthy cells is done by means of a blood examination (Dr R De Greef mentioned above). Applying the Dries diet, which contains several natural antioxidants, can increase that resistance. Anyone wanting to apply ozone therapy should definitely follow the diet.

There are also several other alternative methods that are applied in the fight against cancer. It is very difficult to assess their value, though. Besides, there has not been enough research done regarding the usefulness of these alternative methods. Quite honestly, except for a limited number of foodstuffs, there is nothing at all that seems to have a direct influence on cancer. These other products have been said to influence the defence mechanism, the metabolism or other systems, which means they merely have an indirect influence on the recovery process.

Bio-energetic Readings

Every living organism has a life power that is called bio-energy. This vital energy controls the entire organism. Just as the bio-energy of foodstuffs can be measured, the bio-energetic value of a person can also be measured. We are not talking about a method of diagnosis here, because cancer can only be diagnosed with certainty by means of microscopic examination combined with scans and X-rays and blood analysis. The purpose of the readings is to follow the evolution of the diet. After a few readings we can already tell whether or not the diet is successful. Usually it is possible to notice marked progress every month. A bio-energetic reading is a very important encouragement for a patient, because it not only allows him or her to see the progress for him- or herself, but also expresses the progress in numbers. Initially only the cancer resistance is measured, but afterwards readings are also taken regarding the metabolism, the defence mechanism, the nervous system and separate organs such as the liver, the spleen, the kidneys, etc. The bio-energetic readings allow us to evaluate the improvement of the patient's condition. That improvement has to be confirmed by a hospital examination.

During the initial phase, when the first improvements have been determined, the clinical data do not always manifest themselves yet. That is logical, since it is energy we are measuring. The organism will only start to react once a certain level has been reached. Cancer patients usually follow the evolution with great interest; it encourages them to continue the diet and to apply it even more strictly. Because the values are expressed in numbers, patients can draw up graphs and make comparisons in order to follow their own evolution.

It may be noted that these energetic readings are always analogous to the conclusions of the specialist at the hospital. Several patients make it a habit to drop by for energetic readings before going to their physician for a check-up. If the reading is positive, they can go to their physician with an easy mind, because they already know that the results of their check-up will

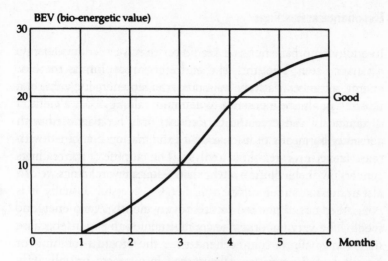

Figure 13 Sample graph of an evolution

also be all right. One of my patients, Jan Peeters, faxed me the following message: 'As you predicted, the X-ray of my bones was even better than that of January. My skeleton is as good as that of a healthy person.' Like many other patients, Jan was surprised to discover that bio-energetic readings are almost always spot on.

Patricia Ooms got breast cancer at the age of 26. Three years later, the cancer had spread to the lungs, one of the hips, the spinal column and the liver. Therapists had given up on Patricia, especially when the chemotherapy did not produce any results, and they discontinued all treatments. An alternative therapist advised her to start applying the Dries diet and at the same time insisted on new chemotherapy. This time the chemotherapy was effective. Patricia's attending physician, who did not know she had been following the Dries diet, was speechless with amazement when he noticed the sudden reversal. In barely 12 months, the c.a. markers dropped from 640 to 31. The cancer had disappeared from her lungs, liver and bones. When Patricia asked her physician about her condition, he answered: 'You are 100 per cent cured.'

Resonance test

In addition to bio-energetic readings, we have also developed a resonance test. The aim of that test is to determine to what extent a cancer patient responds energetically. Experimental research has made it possible to determine the resonance value of a number of cancer patients. Patients with a rather serious or advanced form of cancer reacted to the test with a high resonance (reverse or reciprocal reading). If a patient suffers from cancer, he or she emits on a certain frequency and reacts to the test by means of a resonance.

Energetic readings are linked to wavelength, frequency and speed. The speed is obtained by multiplying the wavelength by the frequency. Resonance means reflection. In effect, the emission of the patient reflects the emission of the test. This happens on the same frequency. The more serious the condition of the patient, the higher the speed on that frequency, which explains the high resonance or the reciprocal reading. As the condition of the patient improves, the speed decreases and the resonance value drops or disappears completely.

As long as there remains a resonance, the first step has to be to dispose of it by means of the diet. When the resonance value has finally been reduced to zero, we can start to think about building up the cancer resistance of the patient. Patients will have a high, an average or a low resonance value. Even though the seriousness of their disease is in the first place determined by means of diagnosis in the hospital, the resonance test offers several advantages for the application of the diet and for counselling. It is the way in which progress is diagnosed.

As soon as the resonance has disappeared completely, further improvements are determined by means of bio-energetic readings. The withdrawal or the absence of a resonance means that the condition is very likely to improve in a favourable way.

Here is a simple explanation. Compare the cancer patient with a drowning person on the high sea, and think of the diet as a lifeboat. The diet gives the drowning person enough strength to swim towards the lifeboat, but that involves a lot of risks. The moment he or she gets into the lifeboat, though, his or her resonance is gone. The second assignment is to try to reach the shore, which does not involve as many dangers. Once the person is ashore, the adventure is over and he or she is declared cured. At that moment, the patient has a very high bio-energetic value. If he or she can maintain that high energetic value by eating and living in a healthy way, there is virtually no chance of relapse.

Both the bio-energetic readings and the resonance test are important means to measure the influence of the diet on the patient. They make it possible for us to follow the evolution of a patient. I have developed these two specific measuring methods myself and, because I have a lot of experience with them, I have a lot of trust in them. The readings are obtained by means of a Lecher antenna, a very complicated measuring instrument. We have also made several attempts to obtain readings by means of electronic instruments, but up to now those readings have not yet been successful. Further, the frequency of the cancer resistance, on which the entire diet is based, is my personal discovery. To prevent abuse, I cannot mention that frequency here; but – as the research advances – I am certainly prepared to cooperate and place my experience and knowledge at other people's disposal. Thus, for now, the readings can only be done in the health centre Avincenna in Genk (Belgium), where I work. There are, however, other ways to measure the evolution of the Dries diet. Every physician, therapist or dietician who is familiar with the Dries diet and bio-energetic readings can assess the improvement. Apart from that, we always take into account the medical record of the attending physician or the hospital.

Results

The fact that this diet has a positive influence on the recovery process has been proven so many times that no one doubts it any more. But still there are those who want to know the exact percentage of patients who have been cured by the diet. After all, people are quite used to thinking in terms of percentages and statistics, and always want to determine their own chance of recovery. But in this case statistics cannot really be established, since the Dries diet gives everyone the same impulses, but with not every patient being capable of taking advantage of those impulses in the same way. The effect of the Dries diet is always individual and depends on dozens of factors, some of which are: the specific features of the tumour, the form of cancer, the location of the tumour, the degree of metastasis, the quality of the defence mechanism, etc. There are also a number of factors we have not yet been able to examine. There are so many aspects that can be of influence. Some patients get a positive prognosis and the disease proves fatal in spite of that. Other patients recover against all odds. Bio-energetic readings allow us to determine the life force of a patient, but we cannot predict a patient's behaviour. Life seems to protect its own secrets. Because cancer is a life-threatening disease, most patients think survival is the only possible result. It is wrong to think that way, however.

If cancer strikes, the best thing to do is to start applying the diet as soon as possible. The result is bound to come, whatever that result may be. And as we have said before, there are dozens of other factors that determine the final result. The Dries diet has to be seen as an important, even unmistakable support of the recovery process. I have mentioned not only patients who managed to conquer their disease, but also patients who did not succeed in doing that. For them, the diet was just as useful. They did not pine away under inhuman conditions, as is often the case. They did not spend their last months surrounded by all kinds of machines and appliances or completely numbed by anaesthetics. They were able to experience their disease in a very conscious way, surrounded by their family, living very intensely from day to day. They were able to bid farewell to life with dignity and serenity. Given the circumstances, that in itself is a laudable result.

A large number of cancer patients would also have recovered

without the diet. People manage to conquer their disease merely by means of regular daily treatments. But those who follow the diet, I believe, are more likely to recover. The recovery process will go by more rapidly and leave less destruction. The diet will also reduce the chance of relapse. The disease will have a more human character and will be easier to bear. It is especially the passive part that the patient usually plays that has such a significant psychological impact on the patient him- or herself and on his or her environment. For a number of patients, the Dries diet did play a decisive part in their recovery. They would never have survived without the diet.

I have already mentioned Patrick Vandenbosch, the man whose oncologist told him he only had three months left to live. Later the oncologist told Patrick that – during his whole career – he had never seen anyone recover from such a tumour. Two years ago, Patrick had to undergo surgery. Unfortunately the surgeons managed to remove only part of the brain tumour. After that, Patrick stayed in hospital and took a number of radiation treatments. He came to see me at the pleading of his despairing wife. We had a long and profound conversation, but I could not promise him much. A month later he visited me again. He told me that he was following the Dries diet very strictly and that he was feeling a lot better. During his third visit I was informed of the great news: a scan had shown that there were no traces of the tumour left. During that same year, Patrick consulted a neuro-surgeon. The neurosurgeon was very satisfied with the results. Another scan confirmed that everything was all right. I received a letter, from which I have copied a fragment:

Last May, I had an appointment with the neurosurgeon, to discuss the results of the scanner examination. The surgeon couldn't find any, not even the slightest trace of relapse. Because the results of the scan and the EEG were very positive, the surgeon decided to reduce the dose of the drug Diphantone. Instead of three times a day, I only have to take a tablet against epilepsy twice a day now. Whereas three months ago the surgeon said it would certainly take five more years for me to recover, he is saying something completely different now. He says that we are on the road to complete recovery, but that it is still too soon to shout victory though. But he does think I'm going to recover, after the operation that was performed one year and three months ago.

In August, I received a second letter from Patrick. It was even more optimistic. Just read the following fragment:

On August 9 I had to take another EEG examination. The result was simply staggering. My last EEG examination had taken place in May, as you know. The neurologist was very formal in his conclusion. He said that this result was comparable to and even better than the result of May. The neurologist was also impressed with the fact that I hadn't had a single epileptic fit since then. The EEG did show that I had been operated on, but it didn't show any kind of relapse or any other kind of additional damage.

After having consulted the neurologist, I still had to consult the neurosurgeon. His decision was just as astounding. In May I had been taking only two tablets of Diphantone a day. Now I only have to take one tablet a day. Within three months, I still have to take a NMR-scan once more and dependent on the result they will decide whether or not I have to continue taking Diphantone.

Now, two years later, Patrick has recovered completely. He no longer has to take medication. He feels excellent, but it has taken him a long time to regain control of his emotions. At a certain point he was so close to death that it was difficult for him to realize that he was not going to die. Now that all of that is behind him, he is cheerful again, enjoying every moment of life with his four children. He realizes that the Dries diet saved his life.

The case of Patrick Vandenbosch is not an isolated one as you can deduce from the numerous examples mentioned earlier. I have often let other patients read the two letters I got from him. It gives them a lot of confidence. Unfortunately, patients seldom write letters. The reason for that is that they usually visit me personally and because I can be reached by telephone every day between 1 and 2pm. And many times physicians do not believe that their patients have recovered in spite of everything, especially when all regular treatments have been discontinued. It is difficult for them to believe in the influence of the Dries diet. Nevertheless, some amazing recoveries can only be attributed to the application of the Dries diet, as several oncologists have confirmed.

Sometimes people ask me on what kind of cancer the Dries diet has a positive influence. Basically, the kind of cancer is not that important. We have achieved positive results with all kinds of cancer. The reader of this book has probably noticed that I often mention recoveries from brain tumours. A brain tumour is generally removed surgically, but in some cases that is not possible. That is why a lot of patients who start applying the Dries diet still have a tumour or a partial tumour. It is in those patients that we can regularly see the tumour disappear. In other patients that is not possible, because the tumour has already been removed completely during surgery.

One cancer patient, Mia Verbeeck, was suffered from an inoperable breast carcinoma. Her condition was very serious and the prognosis was negative. Mia went through some very rough times, but she never lost heart. After she had applied the diet very strictly for 18 months, her physician told Mia that her condition was improving and, shortly after that, that she had recovered. Mia had followed the diet for quite a long time. The diet is usually applied for 3 to 6 months at the most. Another patient, Arlette Coenen, followed it for 13 months: she also suffered from a breast carcinoma, with metastasis in lungs and bones. Arlette's condition was so serious that a nurse kept on telling her: 'Don't fool yourself, you are dying.' It was extremely difficult for Arlette to live between hope and despair, but in the end she came through. After the 13 months, her physician said to her: 'You have been very lucky; you are cured.' Her husband gave the physician a copy of this book and added: 'My wife has been following this diet for thirteen months now. She owes her life to it.' The physician suddenly understood where Arlette's luck had come from: she had worked on it herself. I could mention any of hundreds of similar cases, all equally fascinating and surprising.

But I don't know what else I can do to convince people of the value of this diet. If anyone is confronted with cancer, he or she should not hesitate but should start following the diet immediately. The Dries diet increases the chance of recovery, counterbalances the side-effects of the severe treatments and decreases the chance of relapse.

Conclusion

Cancer still has many other aspects, such as – for example – the influence of cancer on the relatives of the patient, or the influence of cancer on a relationship or on the children of a patient. In a family with a cancer patient, the new problems that arise are often noticed too late. Cancer in children needs to be approached in a different way because it entails a completely different set of problems. Other aspects of cancer are: life after cancer, the fear of relapse, feeling mutilated after an amputation, the social consequences, assistance, palliative care, psychological counselling, self-help groups, etc.

In this book I have tried to pay attention to the practical application of my diet. I have deliberately avoided the food–cancer discussion. From my practical experience with cancer patients, I have tried to introduce the diet and while doing that have pointed out the favourable influence of the diet on the recovery process, the metabolism and the defence mechanism. I cannot emphasize enough that every cancer patient can benefit by applying the diet. It increases the chance of recovery while reducing the influence of the destructive side-effects of chemotherapy or radiotherapy, so that the organism can recover more rapidly.

I admit that not many people are familiar with this new, bio-energetic approach. They are not comfortable with it yet, but as shown in this book, analytical research regarding foodstuffs runs parallel to bio-energetic research. The discovery of phytochemicals in a number of the foodstuffs that are part of my diet irrefutably proves that link. So sceptics should not be too quick in asking for proof, but should first compare the destroyed, cooked food eaten by thousands of cancer patients every day with the fresh, unspoilt food the patients who follow my diet eat. It does not need being a nutritionist to know that there is a big difference. That the results are different too is more than obvious. With our diet, not much is taken away from a cancer patient, only his or her wrong food and wrong lifestyle. In return, we offer the patient a realistic chance of recovery. During a radio broadcast, someone made the following comment: 'If your diet is so good, then why is it not applied in every single hospital?' I would like to answer that question with a saying from Dr Nolfi's book *Living Food*, which is about the influence of raw food on cancer. In her book, Dr Nolfi quotes a famous statement of Goethe: 'Mankind is annoyed because the truth is so simple.' It is just too good to be true, and yet it is the truth. For years, I have worked intensely on the development of this diet, and for years I have been applying it on hundreds of cancer patients and systematically following their evolution. Apart from that, hundreds of other patients have followed the diet without contacting me. Now I am completely convinced that the diet works and that it cannot be compared to any other diet. Because the results are so positive, I consider it my duty to give this diet as much publicity as possible. That way I will be able to contribute to the need of thousands of cancer patients all over the world who are begging for help. Do not search for evidence, they must be told, do not force the government to subsidize research or to acknowledge the results; just apply the diet and see for yourself what the results are. Waste no precious time: grab the opportunity and start today – what good will it do if tomorrow ten famous scientists prove that the diet does work, but the day after tomorrow ten equally famous scientists try to undermine the results with clever arguments: science often *does* works that way. I am counting on everyone who works with cancer patients to help me promote this diet: researchers, oncologists, medical specialists, organizations who wage the war against cancer and especially the numerous self-help groups. Recommend this diet and convince yourself of the results! Your patients will thank you for it. Furthermore, it is my pleasure to help – in any way I can – professionals who are participating in the fight against cancer and who are treating and counselling cancer patients. I am not looking for recognition. My only aim is to contribute to the fight against the growing cancer problem. The Dries diet is a complementary therapy that can be applied simultaneously with the regular treatment without causing any problems. The diet does not entail side-effects or any other dangers. All you have to do is to follow the instructions as they are described here. The Dries diet consists solely of natural foodstuffs that are eaten in an unspoilt way. It does not cause nutritional shortages in the body because it contains sufficient amounts of nutrients and other necessary substances. Moreover, it improves the digestion, the absorption and the metabolism so thoroughly that the need for food decreases. The ingredients of the Dries diet are by nature suitable for the human digestive system, and do not entail any risks. Besides, every patient who applies the Dries diet remains under the supervision of his or her attending physician and follows all the instructions of that physician. The Dries diet is not commercial in any way; apart from the patient who applies it, no one benefits from its application.

After a long experimental phase of closely following the evolution of hundreds of cancer patients, I have more than enough proof and absolute certainty that the Dries diet is a valuable complementary therapy. I am convinced this diet is a blessing for mankind. No one can ignore the positive results of this diet, which up to now no other diet has managed to obtain. That is why we are doing our best to promote this diet all over the world. I will say it once more: 'I believe in miracles because I've seen so many happen.'

Appendix:

A Summary of the Dries Cancer Diet

The Dries cancer diet enjoys an international fame that can only be put down to its surprising results. The medical parameters of the cancer patients who follow this diet evolve favourably within a very short period of time. These patients recover with incredible speed, are barely troubled by the side-effects of chemotherapy or radiotherapy, while their chance of recovery improves considerably. What is the strength of this remarkable diet?

The Dries cancer diet is based on the bio-energetic principle according to which a plant consists of transformed sunlight. On one hand, that sunlight is converted into organic compounds (photosynthesis) and on the other hand it is stored in the DNA, in the form of biophotons. All the components of a foodstuff, like protein, fat, carbohydrates, vitamins, enzymes, colouring agents, flavourings and many other substances should be considered as condensed light energy. We are talking about light energy that has condensed in such a way that it has created substantial structures, while free energy runs the organism in the form of life force. There is an interaction between the bio-energy (free energy), the life force of a foodstuff, and the components of that foodstuff (condensed energy).

Bio-energetic research started with the experiment of the Russian scientist Alexander Gurwitsch (1923) but it wasn't developed until later (1973–1985), by Prof. Dr Popp and his colleagues at the Max Planck Institute in Heidelberg. Popp discovered the biophotons in organisms. He succeeded in measuring their amounts, in making them visible, in determining the degree of order and disorder, in accurately determining the biophoton emission and in developing the biophoton quality analysis, the new method to determine the quality of a foodstuff.

All over the world scientists are working on biophoton research. Especially well known is the research centre of the Tohoku University in Japan. In bio-energetic research, the quality of a foodstuff is not only based on its analytical value (components), but also on its degree of order. This degree of order depends on its ability to retain biophotons in the DNA for a longer period of time. The terms 'order' and 'disorder' are very important, not only as far as the bio-energetic science is concerned, but also in the complementary fight against cancer. Their description is based on the research of Prof. Dr Fröhlich (University of Liverpool) on one hand and the research of Belgian Nobel Prize winner Prof. Dr I Prigogine on the other hand.

The bio-energetic value

The most important contribution of J Dries to the development of his cancer diet is the fact that he managed to distinguish 'cancer resistance' and 'immunity'. Both forms of resistance have a specific frequency, which made it possible for him to discover foodstuffs with a high bio-energetic value, both on the frequency of cancer resistance and on the frequency of immunity and metabolism. His research has proven that a number of fruits have a very high bio-energetic value on the desired frequencies. That is understandable if you know that fruits originate from flowers or blossoms, which – because of their suitable structure – are capable of absorbing vast quantities of biophotons. Furthermore, the degree of improvement (upgrading) of the plant has been found to be decisive. That is why wild berries and tropical fruits are preferred to homegrown fruits. A number of vegetable varieties, mostly those with a delicate structure and those that grow above ground, are also suitable.

The Dries cancer diet consists of ingredients with a high bio-energetic value on the frequency of cancer resistance, metabolism and immunity. The latter is important if the patient is being treated by means of chemotherapy or radiotherapy. A patient who applies the Dries cancer diet receives a direct energy pulse, which increases the electropotential of his or her cells. This means that all processes on all levels will take place more smoothly and especially more intensely, which makes repolarization of the damaged cells possible.

Not only the free energy in the form of biophotons is important. The condensed energy in the form of nutritive and antinutritive components also plays an important part in the recovery process. It is the interaction between both aspects that determines the degree of order. The Dries cancer diet is very easily digestible because it largely consists of watery fruits. Modern anatomy and physiology irrefutably prove that human-kind has the digestive system of a frugivore. Adapting what is eaten to the digestive system not only improves digestion but also leads to a more efficient metabolism. The Dries cancer diet leaves behind remarkably few homotoxins, while its purifying effect is very profound because of an almost perfect sodium–potassium balance and a favourable acid–base balance. Because of this, both the intra- and the extracellular fluid are cleaned, which has a re-straining influence on the formation of cancerogenes. Moreover, possible cancerogenes are secreted more easily or even destroyed.

Because everything is eaten raw, not a single component can be damaged. This is very important for the enzymatic effect. A well-balanced protein supply, in which not only all the essential amino acids are represented, but also all the auxiliary substances such as intact vitamins, active minerals, trace elements and natural antioxidants, makes sure that the diet is complete. Everything is supplied to the organism in nearly perfect pro-portions. That is why someone who is following the diet will not suffer from shortages or from malnutrition. A molecular biologist who works at a nutritional institute and who followed the diet himself for a while, was completely surprised by the change in the pattern of his needs. Once you have switched over to the Dries cancer diet, you will feel more than satisfied, your body weight will remain stable, you will be able to perform better than expected on the physical level and you will be able to regain your health in no time.

The thermodynamic aspect

The strength of the Dries cancer diet is partly hidden in the thermodynamic aspect of water. Water is an essential component of fruit and vegetables, in which it can be found in large quantities. Just as protein has a natural relationship with fat, carbohydrates have a natural relationship with water and the vitamins that can be dissolved in water. Quantitatively, carbohydrates and sugars are the most important components of our food. Apart from protein and fat, they supply the body with a major amount of warmth. That warmth is retained by water. This can be compared to what happens in regions with a maritime climate. What is important about the thermodynamic aspect is that it stabilizes the central temperature by activating the capillaries. Both the organs and the tissues receive more blood, larger quantities of oxygen, warmth and nutrition, while the discharge of homotoxins improves. In the beginning, switching over to the diet can lead to chills, but only until the thermoregulation has adjusted itself.

Nearly all sugars in the Dries cancer diet are simple or double sugars. The diet barely contains complex sugars. The advantage of that is that the sugars are released and converted rather quickly, which leads to a stable blood sugar level and relief of the pancreas. Some patients lose a lot of weight when they switch over to the diet, which forces them to keep on using foodstuffs that contain a lot starch for a slightly longer period of time. The main reason for that is that their disrupted water regulation has not restored itself yet.

Bioactive substances

The Dries cancer diet contains a lot of bioactive substances (secondary plant products or phytochemicals). These are substances with a restraining influence on cancer. We have been paying a lot of attention to bioactive substances these last few years. At the University of Illinois in Chicago they have installed a data bank that contains more than 50,000 publications on bioactive substances in foodstuffs. The National Cancer Institute of the United States has made 50 million dollars available for a research programme that is meant to detect the cancer-restraining influence of secondary plant products in foodstuffs.

The primary nutrients are: protein, fat, carbohydrates, vitamins and minerals. The science of nutrition has already described them elaborately. The secondary plant products are substances that occur only in plants, in very small quantities. They have a healing or pharmacological effect. Because the word 'secondary' sometimes also means 'in the second place' or 'less important', we prefer to speak of 'bioactive substances' or 'phyto-chemicals', because – after all – these products are of major importance to the health of humankind.

Experiments that were carried out between 1985 and 1995 prove that the regular and frequent use of vegetables and fruit has a favourable influence on recovery from certain types of cancer. Each human cell contains genes that make the development of cancer possible, but under normal circumstances that does not happen because of blockades. Sometimes, however, those block-ades are raised by genotoxic carcinogens. Luckily, human kind possesses a cancer resistance, a protective mechanism that fights the effects of carcinogens. The cancer resistance is aided by enzymes in the body and the bioactive substances that are found in food. These substances are capable of repairing defects in the

DNA. The development of a tumour is always supported by promoters. Promoters are substances that can influence the cell regulation. Animal fats, alcohol and food with a high calorific value (like high-protein or high-starch food) are considered promoters.

Food that contains a lot of vitamins and minerals together with bioactive substances is considered an anti-promoter and increases the cancer resistance.

Cancer develops when the bio-energetic value on the frequency of cancer resistance drops in such a way that the enzymatic effect is restrained and the balance between carcinogens and anti-carcinogens, between promoters and anti-promoters is disrupted. Bioactive substances are: carotenoids, phyto-sterin, saponins, glucosinolates, polyphenols, protease-inhibitors, terpenes, phyto-estrogens, sulphides and substances derived from fermented foodstuffs. Because they prevent cancer, the substances that are called 'roughage', like rough fibres, cellulose, pectins etc., are also considered bioactive substances. Apart from their anti-carcinogenic effect, bioactive substances possess numerous other qualities. Bioactive substances are found in fruit, vegetables and fermented products, like yoghurt and sauerkraut. All the presently known foodstuffs that contain bioactive substances are part of the Dries cancer diet.

Research has shown that cooking, baking and stewing causes a serious loss of bioactive substances. Warmth also disrupts the bio-energetic value because it leads to a disintegration of the structure. The Dries cancer diet is a raw food diet and that is mainly why its effects are so favourable.

The Dries cancer diet is a diet that is well ahead of its time. In the beginning of the 1980s, when scientists were in a feverish hurry to discover possible bioactive substances, the Dries cancer diet was developed and tested on hundreds of cancer patients. Now we have found that the diet contains extremely high amounts of bioactive substances. Worldwide research confirms the accuracy of bio-energetic research and largely explains the successful effects of the Dries cancer diet. The favourable results of the Dries cancer diet can be put down not only to the high bio-energetic value on the frequency of cancer resistance, metabolism and immunity of the foodstuffs it contains; the presence of vitamins, minerals and antioxidants; the precise administration of protein and carbohydrates; the favourable sodium–potassium balance; the good acid-base balance and the ample presence of bioactive substances in the diet; but also to the high degree of order. This high degree of order can only be obtained because all the components of the diet are present in correct proportions and because all of them are intact. The secret of the success of the Dries cancer diet lies in its respect for the laws of nature.

Useful Addresses

For advice and counselling

Jan Dries
Avicenna Health Centre
Schepersweg 112
3600 Genk
Belgium
Tel: 32 89 396 169
Fax: 32 89 355 307

For information and professional training:

European Academy for Complementary Health Care
Antwerp-Ghent-Utrecht-Maastricht
Head office
Weg naar As 267
3600 Genk
Belgium
Tel: 32 89 355 246
Fax: 32 89 355 259

Organizations:

The following listing is for information only and does not imply any endorsement, nor do the organizations listed necessarily agree with the views expressed in this book.

AUSTRALASIA

Australian Association for Hospice and Palliative Care
PO Box 1200
North Fitzroy
Victoria 3068
Australia
Tel: 3 486 2666
Fax: 3 482 5094

Australian Cancer Society Inc
153 Dowling Street
Woolloomooloo
New South Wales 2011
Australia
Tel: 2 358 2066
Fax: 2 356 4558

Australian Natural Therapists Association
PO Box 3008
Melrose Park
South Australia 5039
Australia
Tel: 8 297 9533
Fax: 8 297 003

Cancer Society of New Zealand Inc
PO Box 12145
Wellington, New Zealand
Tel: 4 473 6409
Fax: 4 499 0849

New Zealand Natural Health Practitioners Accreditation Board
PO Box 37–491
Auckland
New Zealand
Tel: 9 625 9966

NORTH AMERICA

American Cancer Society
1599 Clifton Road NE
Atlanta
Georgia 30329, USA
Tel: 404 320 3333
Fax: 404 325 0230

American Holistic Medical Association
4101 Lake Boone Trail, Suite 201
Raleigh
North Carolina 27607, USA
Tel: 919 787 5146

Canadian Cancer Society
10 Alcorn Avenue, Suite 200
Toronto
Ontario M4V 3B1, Canada
Tel: 416 961 7223
Fax: 416 961 4189

Canadian Holistic Medical Association
700 Bay Street
PO Box 101, Suite 604
Toronto
Ontario M5G 1Z6, Canada
Tel: 416 0047

National Cancer Institute
Building 31, Room 10A24
9000 Rockville Pike
Bethesda
Maryland 20892 USA
Tel: 301 496 5583
Fax: 301 402 2594

National Coalition for Cancer Survivalship
1010 Wayne Avenue
Silver Spring
Maryland 20910, USA
Tel: 301 650 8868

SOUTHERN AFRICA

Cancer Association of South Africa
PO Box 2000
Johannesburg
South Africa
Tel: 11 616 7662

South Africa Homeopaths, Chiropractors and Allied Professions Board
PO Box 17055
0027 Groenkloof
South Africa
Tel: 12 466 455

UK & EIRE

British Association for Counselling
1 Regent Place
Rugby
Warwickshire CV21 2PJ
England
Tel: 01788 578328

British Association for Cancer United Patients (BACUP)
3 Bath Place
Rivington Street
London EC2A 3JR, England
Tel: (Cancer Information Service freeline)
0800 181199, (Cancer Counselling Service)
0171 696 9000

Bristol Cancer Help Centre
Grove House
Cornwallis Grove
Clifton
Bristol BS8 4PG, England
Tel: 0117 9743216

British Complementary Medicine Association
39 Prestbury Road
Cheltenham
Gloucestershire GL25 2PT
England
Tel: 01242 226770

British Holistic Medical Association
Royal Shrewsbury Hospital South
Shrewsbury
Shropshire SY3 8XF, England
Tel: 01743 261155
Fax: 01743 353 637

Cancer Care Society
21 Zetland Road
Redland
Bristol BS6 7AH, England
Tel: 0117 9427419

CancerLink
17 Britannia Street
London WC1X 8JN
Tel: 0171 833 2451

Cancer Relief Macmillan Fund
Anchor House
15–19 Britten Street
London SW3 3TZ, England
Tel: 0171 351 7811

Cancer Research Campaign
10 Cambridge Terrace
London NW1 4JL, England
Tel: 0171 224 1333
Fax: 0171 487 4310

Childhood Cancer and Leukaemia Link
36 Knowles Avenue
Crowthorne
Berkshire RG11 6DU
Tel: 01344 75 0319

Council for Complementary and Alternative Medicine
179 Gloucester Place
London NW1 6DX, England
Tel: 0171 724 9103
Fax: 0171 724 5330

Counselling Information Scotland
Health Education Board for Scotland
Woodburn House
Canaan Lane
Edinburgh EH10 4SG, Scotland
Tel: 0131 452 8989

Dr Sandra Goodman
Positive Health Publications Ltd
51 Queen Square
Bristol BS1 4LJ

Hospice Information Service
St Christopher's Hospice
51–59 Lawrie Park Road
Sydenham
London SE26 6DZ, England

Imperial Cancer Research Fund
PO Box 123
Lincoln's Inn Fields
London WC2A 3PX, England
Tel: 0171 242 0200
Fax: 0171 269 3262

Institute for Complementary Medicine
PO Box 194
London SE16 1QZ, England
Tel: 0171 237 5165
Fax: 0171 237 5175

Irish Cancer Society
5 Northumberland Road
Dublin 4, Eire
Tel: 1 668 1855
(National Helpline) 1 800 200 700

Marie Curie Cancer Care
28 Belgrave Square
London SW1X 8QG, England
Tel: 0171 235 3325

Rainbow Centre For Children With Cancer and Life-Threatening Illness
PO Box 604
Bristol
Avon BS99 1SW
Tel: 0117 973 0752

Ulster Cancer Foundation
40–42 Eglantine Avenue
Belfast BT96 6DX
Northern Ireland
Tel: 01232 663281
(National freephone helpline) 01232 663439

The Vegetarian Society
Parkdale
Dunham Road
Altringham
Cheshire WA14 4QG
Tel: 0161 928 0793

Glossary

Aetiological: of or relating to aetiology, a) the study of the causes of disease b) the cause of a disease.

Aldehydes: class of organic compounds containing the group -CHO directly joined to a carbon atom.

ALS: abbreviation of Amyotrophic Lateral Sclerosis – lateral sclerosis that is accompanied by atrophy of the motor nuclei of the spinal marrow and the brains and also the muscles that are innervated by them. It is a progressive disease that usually has a fatal outcome.

Amino acids: any of a group of organic compounds containing one or more amino groups.

Anthocyanin: of a class of water-soluable glycosidic pigments, especially those responsible for the red and blue colours in flowers. They are closely related to vitamins E and P.

Anthroposophic diet: a diet according to the anthroposophic principles of Rudolf Steiner. The term 'anthroposophy' relates to Steiner's spiritual and mystical teachings, which often makes use of symbols and is based on the belief that certain creative activities are psychologically valuable, especially for educational and therapeutic purposes.

Antigen: a substance that stimulates the production of antibodies.

Apthae: a fungal growth on the mucous membrane of the mouth and throat, commonly known as thrush.

Brainstem: the stalklike part of the brain consisting of the medulla oblongata, the midbrain and the pons Varolii.

Bio-energy: the life energy that is present in each organism (human, animal, plant and micro-organism). Bio-energy is very similar to light energy (biophotons). The quality of food is determined by the quantity of biophotons it contains and the intensity of those biophotons.

Biophotons: units of light energy.

C.a. markers: substances secreted by cells, found in cells or on cells. These 'tumour markers' can take form as genetic markers (abnormal chromosomes), enzymes, hormones, oncofetal antigens, glycoproteins or tumour antigens on cell surfaces produced in response to tumour growth. They are used as a means of detecting early forms of malignancy, making a prognosis and evaluating the nature of a tumour.

Carcinogen: any substance which produces cancer.

Carcinoma: a type of cancer; a malignant tumour in the glandular epithelium, with a tendency towards infiltrating growth and metastasis.

Carotenoid: any of a group of yellow or red pigments, including carotenes, found in plants and certain animal tissues.

Choline: colourless soluable alkaline substance present in animal tissues.

Cytoplasm: the protoplasm of a cell contained within the cell membrane but excluding the nucleus.

Cytostatics: medication that stops the growth and the reproduction of a tumour. There are two groups: the anti-mitotics (which interfere with mitosis) and the antimetabolites (cytotoxics). In recent years there has been a lot of progress in the science of cytostatics.

Cytotoxic: poisonous to living cells; denoting various drugs used in the treatment of cancer.

Dextrorotatory: of rotation to the right; especially the plane of polarization of plane-polarized light passing through a crystal, liquid or solution, as seen by an observer facing the light.

Diaphane: condensation of cell protoplasm which forms the transparent plasma membrane surrounding a cell.

Dietics: the scientific study and regulation of food intake and preparation.

DNA: deoxyribonucleic acid, which carries genetic information in the chromosomes.

Endogenous: developing or originating within an organism.

Endometrial: pertaining to the endometrium, the mucous membrane which lines the uterus.

Enzyme: any of a group of complex proteins or conjugated proteins that are produced by living cells and act as catalysts in specific biochemical processes.

Epidemiology: branch of medical science concerned with the occurrence, transmission and control of epidemic diseases.

Exogenous: having an external origin.

Free radical: also called a 'superoxide radical' – an active oxygen radical that is created during normal metabolic processes. Disruption of the metabolism can lead to an overproduction of free radicals, which causes damage to the cell membranes. Vitamin C, vitamin B, copper, zinc and selenium can help prevent this.

Homoeopathy: method of treating disease by use of small amounts of a drug that in healthy persons would produce symptoms similar to those of the disease being treated.

Humoral: of or relating to the four humours.

Ketones: a class of organic compounds containing the carbonyl group $=CO$ directly joined to two carbon atoms.

Lecher antenna: an instrument of measurement developed by Schneider, a German engineer, and used to measure microwaves (in gigahertz) emitted by living organisms such as humans and raw food.

Leucocytes: also called white blood cells. These cells are part of the human body's defence mechanism and multiply whenever pathogenic (disease producing) organisms enter the body.

Lipidperoxides: oxidation products of fats involved in the development of ketones and aldehydes.

Metastatis: term applied to the process whereby a malignant disease spreads to other parts of the body, and also to the secondary tumours resulting from this process.

Naturopathy: a method of treating disorders which involves the use of herbs and other naturally grown foods, sunlight and fresh air.

Nolfi Diet: a cancer diet developed by Dr Nolfi (1881–1957) in Denmark. Dr Nolfi suffered from breast cancer; in her diet, she always stressed the importance of raw food, which she called 'living food'.

Oncogenes: any of several genes that when abnormally activated can cause cancer.

Oncology: the study, classification and treatment of tumours.

Palliative: of or relating to something which eases pain but may not necessarily effect a cure.

Palliative radiation treatments: radiation that is applied in order to ease pain, but not necessarily to effect a cure.

Pathological: of or relating to pathology, a term which means a) a branch of medicine concerned with the nature and causes of disease b) the manifestations of disease.

Photosynthesis: the process in which the energy of sunlight is used by organisms, especially plants, to synthesize carbohydrates from carbon dioxide and water.

Phytochemicals: chemical of or relating to phytochemistry, the branch of chemistry concerned with the study of plants, their chemical composition and processes.

Polyunsaturated: relating to a class of animal and vegetable fats, the molecules of which consist of long carbon chains with double bonds. Polyunsaturates do not contain cholestrol.

Serotonin: a compound found in the brain, intestines and blood platelets and which acts as a neurotransmitter, as well as inducing contraction of smooth muscle and vasoconstriction.

Symbiosis: an interdependent relationship between two animal or plant species, or between two groups.

Thermoregulation: regulation of heat, maintenance of heat balance in the body.

Thrombocytes: spherical bodies in the blood which are also known as 'platelets' and which play an important part in the process of coagulation in the blood.

Upgrade: in an agricultural sense, this means to improve crops or livestock by crossing them with a better strain.

Bibliography

F.J. Cleton, *Voeding en kanker*, Samson Stafleu, Alphen aan de Rijn/Brussels, 1984

Dr R. De Greef, *Immunologie*, Arinus, Genk, 1992

Dr P.H.W.A.M. De Veer, *Pleidooi voor Biologische kankerbestrijding*, Bigot & Van Rossum, 1988

Jan Dries, *De Nieuwe Kruidengeneeskunde*, Arinus, Genk, 1991

Jan Dries, *Het Dries-dieet*, Arinus, Genk, 1990

Jan Dries, *Kanker genezen volgens de Dr. Nolfi-therapie*, Nieuw Leven, Arinus, Genk, 1986

Jan Dries, *Voedingstherapie* (Diëten en voedingsadviezen bij kanker), Arinus, Genk, 1990

Prof. Dr I. Kazem, *Inleiding tot de oncologie*, Dekker & van de Vegt, Nijmegen, 1983

Gerhard Leibold, *Krebsangst und Krebs behandeln*, Falken Verlag, Niedernhausen/Ts, 1991

Angelika Meier-Ploegar, *Lebensmittelqualität*, Hartmut Vogtmann (Hrsg.), C.F. Müller Verlag, Karlsruhe, 1991

Fritz-Albert Popp, *Die Botschaft der Nahrung*, Karl F. Haug Verlag, Frankfurt, 1993

Fritz-Albert Popp, *Neue Horizonte in der Medizin*, Karl F. Haug Verlag, Heidelberg, 1983

P. Schauder (Hrsg.), *Ernährung und Tumorenkrankungen*, Karger, Basel, 1991

Index

Page numbers in *italics* refer to the glossary